Raising Commercial Dairy Calves

Editors

R.M. THORNSBERRY
A.F. KERTZ
JAMES K. DRACKLEY

VETERINARY CLINICS OF NORTH AMERICA: FOOD ANIMAL PRACTICE

www.vetfood.theclinics.com

Consulting Editor
ROBERT A. SMITH

March 2022 • Volume 38 • Number 1

ELSEVIER

1600 John F. Kennedy Boulevard • Suite 1800 • Philadelphia, Pennsylvania, 19103-2899

http://www.vetfood.theclinics.com

VETERINARY CLINICS OF NORTH AMERICA: FOOD ANIMAL PRACTICE Volume 38, Number 1
March 2022 ISSN 0749-0720, ISBN-13: 978-0-323-84971-5

Editor: Katerina Heidhausen
Developmental Editor: Axell Ivan Jade M. Purificacion

Veterinary Clinics of North America: Food Animal Practice (ISSN 0749-0720) is published in March, July, and November by Elsevier Inc., 360 Park Avenue South, New York, NY 10010-1710. Subscription prices are $267.00 per year (domestic individuals), $656.00 per year (domestic institutions), $100.00 per year (domestic students/residents), $289.00 per year (Canadian individuals), $686.00 per year (Canadian institutions), $342.00 per year (international individuals), $686.00 per year (international institutions), $100.00 per year (Canadian students), and $165.00 (international students). To receive student/resident rate, orders must be accompanied by name of affiliated institution, date of term, and the signature of program/residency coordinator on institution letterhead. *Clinics* subscription prices. All prices are subject to change without notice. **POSTMASTER:** Send address changes to *Veterinary Clinics of North America*: *Food Animal Practice*, Elsevier Health Sciences Division, Subscription Customer Service, 3251 Riverport Lane, Maryland Heights, MO 63043. Customer Service (orders, claims, online, change of address): Elsevier Health Sciences Division, Subscription **Customer Service, 3251 Riverport Lane, Maryland Heights, MO 63043. Tel: 1-800-654-2452 (U.S. and Canada); 314-447-8871 (ouside U.S. and Canada). Fax: 314-447-8029. E-mail: journalscustomerservice-usa@elsevier.com (for print support); journalsonlinesupport-usa@elsevier.com (for online support).**

Reprints. For copies of 100 or more, of articles in this publication, please contact the Commercial Reprints Department, Elsevier Inc., 360 Park Avenue South, New York, NY 10010-1710. Tel.: 212-633-3874; Fax: 212-633-3820; E-mail: reprints@elsevier.com.

Veterinary Clinics of North America: Food Animal Practice is covered in *Current Contents/Agriculture, Biology and Environmental Sciences, MEDLINE/PubMed (Index Medicus), and Excerpta Medica.*

Contributors

CONSULTING EDITOR

ROBERT A. SMITH, DVM, MS
Diplomate, American Board of Veterinary Practitioners; Veterinary Research and
Consulting Services, LLC, Greeley, Colorado, USA; Veterinary Research and Consulting
Services, LLC, Stillwater, Oklahoma, USA

EDITORS

R.M. THORNSBERRY, DVM, MBA
Mid America Veterinary Consulting, Richland, Missouri, USA

A.F. KERTZ, PhD
Diplomate, American College of Animal Nutrition; ANDHIL LLC, St Louis, Missouri, USA

JAMES K. DRACKLEY, PhD
Professor, Animal Sciences, University of Illinois, Urbana, Illinois, USA

AUTHORS

PAMELA R.F. ADKINS, DVM, MS, PhD
Department of Veterinary Medicine and Surgery, University of Missouri, Columbia,
Missouri, USA

JONATHON L. BECKETT, PhD
Beckett Consulting, Fort Collins, Colorado, USA

CHRISTOPHER C.L. CHASE, DVM, MS, PhD
Diplomate, American College of Veterinary Microbiologists; Professor, Department of
Veterinary and Biomedical Sciences, South Dakota State University, Brookings, South
Dakota, USA

DANIEL B. CUMMINGS, DVM
Professional Services Veterinarian, Boehringer Ingelheim Animal Health USA Inc

TAMARA GULL, DVM, PhD, ACVM, ACVPM
Diplomate, American College of Veterinary Internal Medicine (Large Animal); Associate
Clinical Professor, Section Head, Bacteriology/Mycology, Veterinary Medical Diagnostic
Laboratory, University of Missouri CVM, Columbia, Missouri, USA

JAMES GROTHE, BS
Agriculture Education, University of Minnesota, Kent Nutrition Group Strategic Sales
Account Manager, Ruminant Specialist

A.F. KERTZ, PhD
Diplomate, American College of Animal Nutrition; ANDHIL LLC, St Louis, Missouri, USA

RICH LARSON, DVM, PhD
Laramie, Wyoming, USA

NATHAN F. MEYER, MS, MBA, PhD, DVM
Senior Professional Services Veterinarian, Boehringer Ingelheim Animal Health USA Inc, Affiliate Faculty, Department of Clinical Sciences, Colorado State University, Fort Collins, Colorado, USA

BART PARDON, DVM, PhD
Department of Internal Medicine, Reproduction and Population Medicine, Faculty of Veterinary Medicine, Ghent University, Merelbeke, Belgium

SCOTT E. POOCK, DVM
Diplomate, American Board of Veterinary Practitioners; Associate Extension Veterinarian, Animal Science and Research Center, University of Missouri, Columbia, Missouri, USA

DAVID RENAUD, DVM, PhD
Department of Population Medicine, Ontario Veterinary College, University of Guelph, Guelph, Ontario, Canada

RANDY W. ROSENBOOM, MS
Kent Nutrition Group, Estherville, Iowa, USA

DOUGLAS L. STEP, DVM, DACVIM
Professional Services Veterinarian, Boehringer Ingelheim Animal Health USA Inc

R.M. THORNSBERRY, DVM, MBA
Mid America Veterinary Consulting, Richland, Missouri, USA

DAVE WOOD, MBA
Director of Sales and Technical Support, Animix, Juneau, Juneau, Wisconsin, USA

Contents

> The use of beef bulls on dairy cattle has increased in the last 6 years. In fact, beef semen sales have more than doubled. Dairyman needs to capture real value for the beef on dairy cross calf, selection of beef sires that produce offspring that complement dairy cattle are needed, not simply the cheapest black bull in the tank. Those beef sires should be selected on calving ease, ribeye area, marbling, feed efficiency, fertility, polled, and an industry preference for black hided. Even more important, the use of beef on dairy has allowed dairy producers to manage replacement animal inventories.

> Vaccination is an important component for the prevention and control of disease in calves. Too often vaccines are viewed as a catch-all solution for management and nutrition errors; the "best" vaccine can never overcome these deficiencies. Proper vaccination in the young calf and developing heifer is the key to long-term development of a productive dairy cow. To actually immunize animals, animals must be able to respond to vaccines, which is dependent on the level of animal husbandry. Each vaccine program needs to be designed based on animal flow, actual "disease" threats, and labor on the farm.

> There are a variety of feeding programs that can meet the goal of doubling calf birth weight at the end of 2 months of life. Feeding programs need to take into account the inverse relationship between mil/milk replacer and starter intakes. Water is the most essential nutrient needed in the greatest quantity by calves. Water is consumed at about 4 times dry matter intake and should be fed warm during cold weather. Water and starter should be fed sooner and forage later than the 2014 NAHMS data indicate US dairy producers are doing.

> The development of modeling concepts with the 2001 NRC (National Research Council Nutrient Requirements of Dairy Cattle represented a

big step toward understanding and applying the underlying mechanisms associated with young calf growth. Factors such as the plane of nutrition being provided (protein and energy), breed and environmental stressors impact calf growth. Investigation into delivering the proper amounts of energy and protein through the liquid and dry feeds to optimize growth needs to continue as well as further defining the most effective means to transition from the nonruminant to ruminant phase while minimizing post-weaning lag.

The transition for the calf from the milk-feeding phase to the grouping and dry feed feeding phase is the second most difficult time for a calf, with the most difficult life phase being parturition and the first day of life. Reducing these stress factors directly relates to reduced health problems and better performance during subsequent life phases. This review will discuss some of the key management factors associated with achieving maximum production potential for the commercial dairy calf.

Surplus male dairy calves experience significant health challenges after arrival at the veal and dairy beef facilities. To curb these challenges, the engagement of multiple stakeholders is needed starting with improved care on some dairy farms and better management of transportation. Differing management strategies are also needed if calves arrive at veal and dairy beef facilities under poor condition.

Raising young dairy calves presents many challenges for producers and veterinarians including losses attributable to BRD. This article will discuss several key concepts for practitioners to consider when applying evidence-based medicine for the control and treatment of BRD in young dairy calves. The authors review BRD complex, provide considerations for diagnostic approaches, and discuss research associated with the control and treatment of BRD.

Although diarrhea in dairy calves is common, it is not always due to bacteria. *Escherichia coli, Salmonella,* and *Clostridium perfringens* are the most commonly implicated bacteria, but an etiologic diagnosis should be sought before specific treatment is instituted. Nonspecific treatment such as fluid, electrolyte, and nutritional support should be accomplished while diagnostics are pending. Antimicrobials should not be a first-line therapy for calf diarrhea. Control measures are discussed.

Cryptosporidiosis is a common cause of diarrhea among preweaned dairy calves. In the United States, the most common species of Cryptosporidium found in dairy calves is Cryptosporidium parvum, an important zoonotic species. Cryptosporidiosis is spread by fecal-oral transmission. Calves begin shedding the oocysts as early as 2 days of age, with peak shedding occurring at 14 days of age. Diarrhea generally starts 3 to 4 days after ingestion of the oocysts. Risk factors for the disease include large dairy farms, summer months, feeding of milk replacer, and early feeding of starter grain. Concrete flooring and appropriate cleaning of feeding utensils decreases the risk of disease.

 Video content accompanies this article at http://www.vetfood. theclinics.com.

CMR's should be composed primarily of milk proteins, lactose as the sole carbohydrate source, lipids composed of edible grade tallow or lard with consideration for medium-chain fatty acids derived from coconut oil that mimic those in milk fat and adequate vitamin and mineral nutrition. Spray-dried bovine plasma provides antibodies shown to reduce diarrhea and calf mortality and to effectively replace a significant portion of milk protein in the diet. Whole milk pasteurization must be intensely monitored to ensure it is consistently wholesome. Milk is deficient in vitamins and trace minerals.

Rumen development from weaning, 200 pounds (91 kg) to 400 pounds (181.2 kg), is critical and depend on proper papillae development. Papillae development is tied to propionic and butyric acid production in the rumen, and this favors a diet based on concentrate. Forage intake produces acetic acid, which does not promote papillae development. Previous research illustrates that although increasing forage intake as a percentage of the dry matter diet increases rumen size, it shows a reduction in papillae length compared with diets containing a lower percentage of forage and a higher percentage of concentrate intake.

VETERINARY CLINICS OF NORTH AMERICA: FOOD ANIMAL PRACTICE

SERIES OF RELATED INTEREST

Veterinary Clinics: Equine Practice
https://www.vetequine.theclinics.com/

THE CLINICS ARE NOW AVAILABLE ONLINE!
Access your subscription at:
www.theclinics.com

Preface

Raising Commercial Dairy Calves

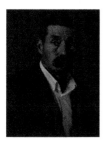 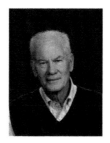 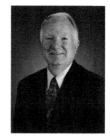

R.M. Thornsberry, DVM, MBA   A.F. Kertz, PhD   James K. Drackley, PhD

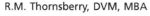

Editors

Raising commercially acquired dairy calves is a multifaceted business. This issue addresses clinically important practices for commercial replacement dairy heifer raising operations, dairy beef operations, and white veal and "rose or pink" veal operations. It also addresses their transitional phases of production up to 180 kg (400 lb) of body weight. While each of these production systems has varied nuances, basic management and veterinary medical clinical practices apply. These industries are relatively small in number and privately owned. Acquiring access to production data to evaluate growth rates, daily gain, feed efficiency, disease prevalence, diagnostic reports, or currently utilized protocols is difficult. There is an industry-acquired vocabulary that may be foreign to many food animal veterinary practitioners. These industries are inundated with proprietary product sales requiring veterinary evaluation.

The breeds of dairy beef calves raised commercially have changed dramatically in the last three years (2018-2021). The use of sexed semen resulted in an overproduction of replacement dairy heifers. Dairy producers then switched breed types to composite breed semen to produce a crossbred dairy beef composite calf that was black in color. It has literally become difficult to acquire a load of purebred Holstein dairy beef calves in this new business climate. The meat-packing industry began docking purebred dairy beef calves as much as $US15 to $US20 per 45 kg (100 lb) of live weight. These changing business dynamics resulted in a shift to breed dairy replacement heifers and commercial dairy cows to beef breed bulls. The resulting composite breed dairy calves are literally transforming a previously well-established dairy beef industry. These dairy industry adaptations bring new challenges to the food animal practitioner and the commercial dairy calf raiser.

Commercial dairy calf raisers have little control of calf handling, management, or colostrum provision prior to calf procurement and arrival to their facility. Dairy beef calves, because of their value or perceived value, often receive little to no colostrum before sale. In the United States, death loss for replacement dairy heifers is

Vet Clin Food Anim 38 (2022) ix–x
https://doi.org/10.1016/j.cvfa.2021.12.001
0749-0720/22/© 2021 Published by Elsevier Inc.

documented by the National Animal Health Monitoring System (NAHMS; USDA) survey data to be 6% up to 24 hours of age and another 6% up to weaning. Death loss for replacement dairy heifers from weaning to 225 kg (500 lb) is an additional 6.7%. Death loss data for dairy beef and veal calf operations are difficult to acquire separately, but a European study of 5853 head of Belgian white veal calves found the death loss to be 5.7% up to 3 weeks in facility. These numbers clearly illustrate the need for clinical intervention by food animal veterinarians with knowledge and experience.

It is the desire of the guest editors of this issue, Raising Commercial Dairy Calves, that the information revealed will equip food animal practitioners who seek out and provide practical consulting services to dairy calf raisers in their practice areas. The article authors, through their many years of subject application, will offer the readers a practical source of quickly referenced practice ability. Although the number of dairy cattle operations has been reduced by 41% since 1995 (NAHMS), the increased animal facility population density of the remaining dairy cattle operations makes the knowledge in this issue invaluable to a new or expanding veterinary practice. The owners and managers of today's commercial dairy calf operations have high expectations for the veterinarians they have sought out for a veterinary client-patient relationship.

R.M. Thornsberry, DVM, MBA
Mid America Veterinary Consulting
Richland, MO 65556, USA

A.F. Kertz, PhD
ANDHIL LLC
9909 Manchester Road #366>
St. Louis, MO 63122, USA
www.andhil.com

James K. Drackley, PhD
Animal Sciences
University of Illinois
3208 Fawn Hill Court
Urbana, IL 61802, USA

E-mail addresses:
rthornsberry53@gmail.com (R.M. Thornsberry)
andhil@swbell.net (A.F. Kertz)
jimdrackley@gmail.com (J.K. Drackley)

Changing Demographics of the Commercial Dairy Calf Industry: Why Use Beef on Dairy?

Scott E. Poock, DVM[a],*, Jonathon L. Beckett, PhD[b]

KEYWORDS

• Commercial dairy calves • Beef X dairy • Heifer inventory

KEY POINTS

- The use of beef bulls on dairy cattle has greatly increased in the last 5 to 6 years.
- To capture real value for the beef on dairy cross calf, selection of beef sires that produce offspring that complement dairy cattle are needed, not simply the cheapest black bull in the tank.
- Beef sires should be selected on calving ease, ribeye area, marbling, feed efficiency, fertility, polled, and an industry preference for black hided.
- The use of beef on dairy has allowed dairy producers to manage replacement animal inventories.

INTRODUCTION

There has been a drastic change in the demographics of the commercial dairy industry in the last 5 to 6 years. What was once considered a last resort option is now part of strategic breeding programs on dairy farms. That option is utilization of beef sires on dairy cattle. The choice of beef sire cannot simply be the cheapest black bull that is in the tank, but a bull that produces offspring that meet the requirements of the feeder and packer while still profiting the dairy producer.

The industry has arrived at this point where there are excess heifers on dairy farms partly due to increased fertility along with the use of sexed semen. This excess can lead to the financial burden of raising the cost of developing replacements. Historically, dairy farmers kept every dairy heifer as a replacement, as a heifer should have the best genetics in the herd. On the other hand, if a beef on dairy animal is born on the farm, it is usually sold early in its life. Thus, by using more beef sires, less replacement animals are developed, which leads to cost savings.

[a] S133C Animal Science and Research Center, University of Missouri, Columbia, MO 65211, USA;
[b] Beckett Consulting, 1281 E Magnolia Street, D137, Fort Collins, CO 80524, USA
* Corresponding author.
E-mail address: poocks@missouri.edu

Vet Clin Food Anim 38 (2022) 1–15
https://doi.org/10.1016/j.cvfa.2021.11.001
0749-0720/22/Published by Elsevier Inc.

Historical Perspective

Historically, beef bulls have been used on dairy farms for several reasons. A producer might have chosen to use an Angus or Hereford bull to breed their heifers because of smaller calves and calving ease. Some producers, who were planning on getting out of milking cows, might breed their herd to beef bulls to start a beef herd. Another reason was to use beef on the "problem breeders."

Dairy producers would often use a beef sire on problem breeders. This is a common strategy in today's industry as well.[1] The thought was that this cross would increase hybrid vigor of the resulting embryo/fetus, thus increasing the chance of a pregnancy. Although historic data were not able to be found, current conception rates of beef sires on dairy are available on many farms and will be mentioned later.

Many producers of the past viewed the use of beef bulls as an alternative to Holstein bulls for ease of calving. The more commonly used breeds were Angus (**Fig. 1**) and Hereford. In 1980, 14% of Holstein bull calves were born with difficulty, and over the next 20 years, it only improved 3%.[2] In 2003, sire calving ease for Holsteins began to be incorporated into Net Merit (NM$), and stillbirth was added to the sire summary in 2006.[2] By 2014, the incidence of difficult births for Holstein bull calves had dropped to 5%, so genetic selection has made progress.[2] This improvement within the Holstein breed has put pressure on the beef sires that are used for beef on dairy to be easy calving.

Some dairy producers who find themselves wanting to stop milking cows, and yet retain the farm, have either chosen to raise replacement heifers or breed their dairy animals to beef to form a basis of a beef herd. In the early 1970s, this strategy was used with the newly introduced Continental beef breeds (Simmental, Limousin, Gelbvieh, etc.).

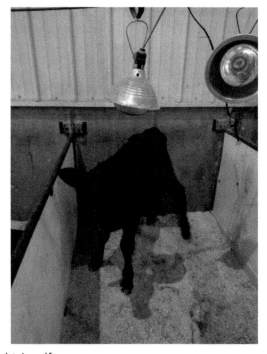

Fig. 1. Angus x Holstein calf.

As can be seen, beef semen sales dating back to 1980 have risen drastically in the last 5 years (**Figs. 2** and **3**). Although some dairymen were using beef on dairy for many years, there was not a tremendous change until recently. In 2018, beef semen sales crossed the 4 million units sold mark for the first time.[3]

Current Situation

Although beef sales are often considered a by-product on dairy farms, they are actually a cash flow source for dairy farms.[4] Therefore, dairy farmers should also be known as beef producers. Recent figures show dairy herds now make up 20.5% to 22.7% of the beef produced in the United States.[5]

Regarding male calves produced on dairy operations, the value of those produced from beef sires is of greater value than full dairy.[4] There are many stories of Jersey bull calves costing a producer for selling them at local livestock auctions rather than receiving a payment.

Owing to this greater value of the beef on dairy animals and the reduced demand by the packing industry of cattle from straight dairy genetics, the trend of using beef genetics has greatly increased, and it is not confined only to the United States, but in other countries as well. Donagh Berry, Director of VistaMilk SFI Centre, and Teagasc geneticist, County Cork, Ireland, has published several articles on this subject. He was able to mine the Irish database and found one-third of matings within the dairy cattle industry were to beef bulls.[6,7]

Through the years, the question of the subsequent performance of the cow after carrying a beef sired animal has been raised by some. Donagh Berry's research was able to evaluate several performance parameters by looking at the cow's lactation after they either had a dairy sired calf (Holstein-Friesian) or a beef sired calf. The article looked at milk/component production as well as milk quality and fertility.[6,7]

The Irish cows that had a beef sired calf produced 50 kg (110 pounds) less milk and had a minor increase in somatic cell count (SCC). However, even though these differences were statistical, economically they would not impact profitability. Specifically, the loss of 110 pounds of milk would amount to ~$17.80 in the United States. This

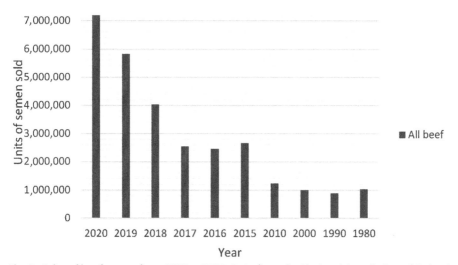

Fig. 2. Sales of beef semen from 1980 to 2020. Data from the National Association of Animal Breeders (NAAB).

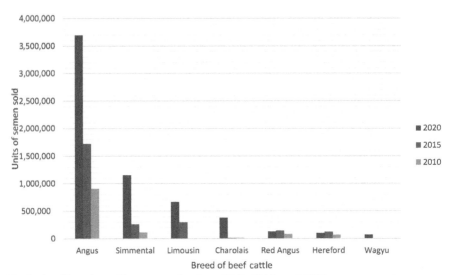

Fig. 3. Beef breed-specific semen sales from 2010, 2015, and 2020.

is considerably less than the more than $100 difference between a dairy calf versus beef calf that is sold.[6,7] Components and reproduction were not affected by the sire of the calf.[6,7]

Interest in beef on dairy calves has increased because of several reasons. First, the improved reproduction of the dairy herd (**Table 1**) has led to increased numbers of re-placements (separate from the use of sexed semen). Once a herd reaches pregnancy rates greater than 18%, farms begin to have excess numbers of heifers in their inventories.[8]

The second reason for the use of beef on dairy is exploitation of potential hybrid vigor effects of the embryo and/or fetus.[4] Thirdly, herd expansion in some countries has curtailed, so more heifer replacements are not necessary.[4] Fourth, the use of sexed semen on the superior dairy animals allows a dairy farmer to produce replace-ments from these matings.[4] Fifth, using beef on dairy creates an alternate cash flow for

Table 1
Improved reproductive parameters from 3 dairy herds from early 2000s until 2021

Reproduction parameters	Herd1 2021	Herd1 2003	Herd2 2021	Herd2 2003	Herd3 2021	Herd3 2006
Heat detection rate	58	65	62	44	61	36
Pregnancy rate	28	18	25	14	22	8
Pregnant first 21 d	27	22	36	16	30	9
% Pregnant by 150 DIM	87	64	79	66	71	47
Average days to first bred	82	61	67	82	74	105
Average days open	112	131	113	129	127	187
Calving interval	12.9	13.2	13	14.1	13.4	14.9
AI conception rate	48	26	40	31	37	24
% of herd pregnant	56	36	54	44	53.2	45

the farm.[4,9] Sixth, there is a growing market for beef on dairy calves.[4] Seventh, there are widely available and extensively proven easy-calving beef bulls.[4] The various breed association and the Integrated Genetic Solutions (IGS) databases have made calving ease Expected Progeny Differences (EPDs and equivalent to dairy's PTA,Predicted Transmitting Ability) much more reliable. Finally, there are increased consumer concerns with the veal industry.[4] As most beef on dairy animals around the globe are grown for more than a year of age before slaughter, this improves the consumer's perception of allowing an animal to live longer.[4] The calves are usually raised as wet calves until 8 to 10 weeks of age, similar to their straight dairy counterparts, then go to a grower before finishing at a feed yard.[4] Harvesting then occurs when the animals are 16 to 18 months of age.[4]

There is a need for the various segments of this industry to work with a veterinarian on protocols that meet animal welfare standards regarding castrating, dehorning (preferably using homozygous Polled beef sires), vaccinating, implant strategies, weaning (should be comparable to their dairy mates), desired weight at various stages, and colostrum management (similar to dairy herdmates).

Many producers have simply sent the resulting beef on dairy calves through normal marketing chains as their dairy counterparts. However, Chip Kemp (American Simmental Association) recommends retaining ownership through slaughter. Selling the animal any time before harvest, someone along the marketing chain is going to try to discount the product.[9] Details on some of the banded programs are covered later in the article.

Heifer Inventory Management

For most of the US Dairy industry history, dairy producers kept every dairy heifer born on the farm. This was regardless of the genetic merit of that heifer. It was assumed that a heifer had improved genetics over its dam. With the decline of fertility within the dairy industry from the 1970s to early 2000s, often there was still a failure to produce enough replacements for annualized turnover rates of 30% to 35%.[10]

However, with improved cow comfort, transition cow management, nutrition, and reproductive management, there is now an abundance of replacements.[10] Add on the use of sexed semen and the result is excess number of heifers.[10]

It should be noted that the grazing and organic dairy farm community have tended to only keep the number of heifers needed to maintain herd size. A breeding strategy used to mate the cows is to AI for a set period and then turn in beef bulls for cleanup. In New Zealand, the use of Hereford bulls to distinguish the switch is common (ie, white face in the calves). Confinement-type dairy farms are now following similar strategies.

However, owing to the cost of raising replacements, it is not always economical to rear every heifer calf, so inventory mitigation practices are useful. Current costs of raising a heifer until she enters the milking herd range from $1700 to 2400.[10] On the other hand, springing heifer prices are only around $1300.[10] Often heifer raising is the most overlooked and undermanaged area of a dairy farm.[11] It typically accounts for 15% to 20% of milk production costs.[11] Heifer raising costs typically is the second or third largest component of the production costs after feed (biggest cost) and labor.

Things to consider when deciding heifer inventory management are as follows: (1) which animals to breed with sexed semen, (2) which dairy calves to raise for replacements, (3) which cows to cull, (4) possible use of beef semen, and (5) whether to use genomic testing.[12]

Culling of the lactating herd is the primary driver of determining the number of heifers needed for replacements. However, calf mortality and disease, fertility of heifers, and elective culling of replacements play a factor in the number of replacements needed.[10] Another way of evaluating the needs for the number of heifers is by simply determining cull rate, heifer cull rate, live heifer inventory, future calvings per month, and finally predicting heifers born per month.[13]

Several spreadsheets have been developed to estimate the number of heifers needed to be born each month to maintain a farm's herd size. These vary from simple to very complex. Most of the AI studs will work with a producer to help establish a program. **Table 2** is an example of the output from a spreadsheet developed by the University of Missouri.

Genomic testing has been around since 2009.[12] Producers have begun to use this type of testing to determine which heifers to raise and which animals to breed to dairy versus beef. Genomic testing works best when combined with the use of sexed semen, that is, breed the best females to have female replacements.[12] Even though the youngest heifers should have the "best" genetics, using DNA testing has shown that this is not always true. Analysis of the genomic testing at the University of Missouri Foremost Dairy revealed that not all heifers have better DNA than their dam (**Fig. 4**).

Similarly, keeping a cow longer will lead to higher productivity and a greater chance of recouping the investment of raising the animal. It is generally accepted that a dairy cow does not return the investment of raising her until late in her second lactation. Likewise, older animals produce more milk than younger animals (**Table 3**).

Another area of dairy management that has improved that affects replacement needs is health of the dairy heifers. The dairy industry has seen improvement by decreasing both morbidity and mortality of replacements. From the 2007 NAHMS report to the 2014 report, there was a decrease from 7.8% mortality in preweaned heifers to 5%. The newest version of the Dairy Calf and Heifer Association's Gold Standards dropped the goal of preweaning death loss from 5% to 3% to continue to set goals that improve the industry.

Strategies for use of beef on dairy.

To begin with, the industry has seen that cows that have lower SCC and higher milk solids (production) are less likely to be bred to beef sires.[4] A female that has had multiple services is more likely to be bred with beef semen.[6] Likewise, an older animal is more likely to be serviced with beef semen.[6,14] If genetic merit is factored into the

Table 2
Estimation of the number of heifers needed to maintain herd size with cost savings compared to current numbers of herd replacements

Herd size	1000
Cost of raising heifer to calving	$1500
Age at first calving	23
Cull rate	38
Noncompletion rate	8
Calving interval	13.1
% of calves born that are heifers	56
Current number of heifers being born on farm per year	535
Number of heifers needed to maintain herd size on an annual basis	393
Per month	33
Excess number of heifers	122
Cost of extra heifers	$45,868.29

Input data in the yellow cells.

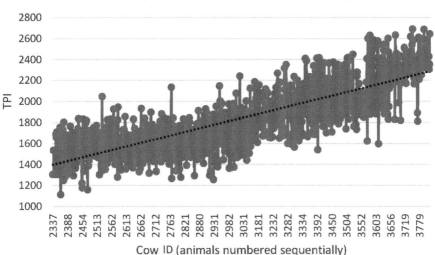

Fig. 4. Total Performance Index (TPI) from Holstein cattle at the University of Missouri's Foremost Dairy. The x-axis has the number of the individual animal with the youngest animals toward the right side of the graph. New animals are numbered sequentially. The y-axis is the GTPI. (Genomic Total Performance Index)

decision, cows with lower merit are more likely to be bred to a beef sire.[6] In situations where the price of a beef on dairy calf is higher, fertility is improved, and/or sexed semen is used along with genomic testing and selection for improved productive life, the benefits of using beef sires are desirable.[15] The changing value premium for the crossbred calf may affect the decision to use beef.[12]

Examples of strategic use of beef on dairy.

Some of the above herds use sexed semen and some do not. However, the strategy of breeding the superior genetic animals in the herd with sexed semen and all others to beef has become popular and is used within the industry.[15]

Table 3
Production from a 1000 cow dairy of the various lactation groups for their average milk production in 305 d

Lactation Group	Pct	Count	M305 (Pounds)
1	33	343	24,657
2	26	270	30,286
3	40	417	31,472
Total	100	1030	28,896

In this situation, the average first lactation produces 78% as much milk in 305 d as the mature cows

WHAT TYPE OF BEEF BULL TO USE?

A survey by Halfman and Sterry revealed that the highest percentage (51%) of producers chose beef semen based on cost.[14] However, the producer should not simply use the cheapest beef semen they can find.

Sixty-two percent of those answering the survey used Angus semen. Another published paper reported 95.4% of beef semen used on dairy was from Angus bulls.[15] Another 18% of those answering the question used Simmental or SimAngus semen along with 18% using Limousin or LimFlex semen.

Central Sands Dairy, which is predominantly Jersey cattle, uses homozygous polled black Gelbvieh bulls to achieve small birthweights, positive growth, and improved carcass parameters.[16] The resulting calves have graded Choice with 13% being Prime with 75% yield grades of 1 or 2.[16]

Some dairymen will use certain breeds of beef cattle out of curiosity for the resulting offspring. For example, a dairy in Wisconsin has used some Brahman (**Fig. 5**). On the other hand, grazing herds in New Zealand will use Hereford clean up bulls to tell which calves are beef sired versus dairy sired (**Fig. 6**).

Continuing with the survey results, 44% of producers chose beef bulls based on calving ease. There are delineated differences in calving ease, perinatal mortality, and gestation length between beef breeds when mated to dairy animals.[4] Angus and Hereford calving ease, when mated to Holstein cattle, is very much similar to Holstein bulls used.[4] However, several of the branded programs (discussed later in the article) are using other breeds and/or composites with emphasis on calving ease.

Similarly, 49% of dairy producers chose beef bulls based on conception rate. Conception rate of Angus bulls is comparable to Holstein bulls, whether to cows or

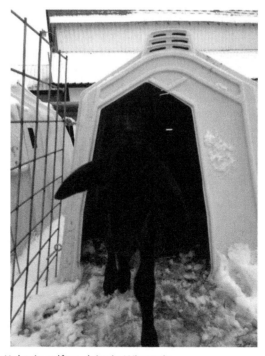

Fig. 5. Brahman x Holstein calf on dairy in Wisconsin.

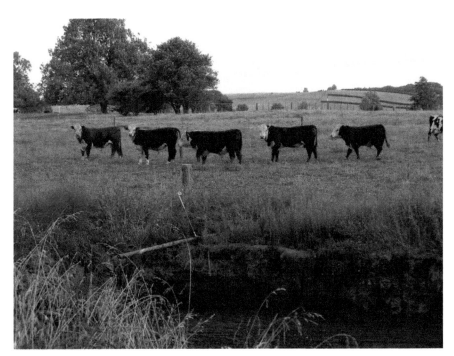

Fig. 6. Hereford bulls being used on a pasture-based herd in New Zealand.

heifers.[15] It should be noted that the Angus sires were used less on first service animals than Holstein sires.[15] However, looking at actual farm data, many farms are not realizing increased conception rates with beef sires (**Tables 4–7**, as examples). This can be partially explained by the use of beef sires on "problem" breeders. However, comparing first service rates from the farms from the examples, Holstein sires still have an advantage.

Finally, the survey indicated that producers had received discounts for heifers (53%), not solid black in color (53%), and horns (17%).[14] Berry and colleagues 2019 developed a breeding index for the Irish dairy industry which looked at the following criteria: (1) direct calf difficulty, (2) direct gestation length, (3) calf mortality, (4) feed intake, (5) carcass merit (carcass weight, conformation, and fat), (6) docility, and (7) polled. Several of the branded programs are developing similar indexes.

Regarding the carcass of dairy animals, they are lighter than those originating from beef herds.[17] It is well accepted that Jersey cattle have light carcass weights. Holstein

Table 4			
This herd determines rank of the cows based on NM$ and then breeds the bottom 25% to beef sires			
Breed	Conception Rate	Total	% of Total Breedings
Holstein	38	356	75
SimAngus	30	114	24
Totals	36	474	100

Table 5
This herd only began using beef in the spring of 2020

Breed	Conception Rate	Total	% of Total Breedings
Holstein	43	2681	73
Angus	36	839	23
Limousin	35	149	4
Totals	41	3669	100

They look at week 6 milk to determine whether a cow will be bred to dairy or beef. If the cow is in the bottom 20% for production at week 6, then she is bred to beef. Likewise, after the 3rd service, most cows will be bred to beef

Table 6
This herd has chosen to breed first calf heifers with sexed semen and a majority of older cows with beef

Breed	Conception Rate	Total	% of Total Breedings
Holstein	38	3904	41
SimAngus	33	5727	59
Totals	35	9631	100

Although, older cows deemed as a high producer will be bred to sexed semen (~25% of older cows)

Table 7
This herd uses production data along with parent PTA to determine the bottom one-third of the herd which are bred to beef sires

	Bottom One-Third of Herd Bred to Beef		
Breed	Conception Rate	Total	% of Total Breedings
Limousin	44	572	31
Holstein	52	1283	69
Totals	49	1859	100

carcasses are longer than other breeds.[9,18] The difference in dressing percent is due to dairy-type animals having more bone, larger viscera, and less muscle.

Beef on dairy carcasses tend to be fatter than straight dairy animals.[4] The industry tends to agree that the dressing percentage of dairy animals is inferior to that of beef animals.[18] Once again, the dairy animal has dressing percentage in the high 50s and low 60s in comparison with beef in the mid 60s.[9]

Dairy breeds historically had better marbling than the average beef breeds. However, this trend is not true today, as the beef industry has bred slaughter steers to produce higher quality grades.[9] Jersey cattle have fat that tends to be more yellow than other breeds.

Dairy breeds need improvements in the shape and size of the ribeye to appear more like a beef animal. Specifically, the dairy animal's ribeye tends to be "narrower" and "longer" than a beef animal.[9] Therefore, within the packing plant, the dairy carcasses can be relatively easily identified and discounted.[9]

Beef on Dairy Branded Programs

The HOLSim program (**Fig. 7**) began in 2018 with joint collaboration between the Holstein and Simmental associations. Data so far show the HOLSim steers gaining in the low 3 lb/d (1.4 kg) and converting 6.2 to 6.5 lb (2.8–3 kg) of feed per pound of gain. The carcasses have been greater than 80% choice or greater with very few yield grade 4. There is lot of datum coming through the IGS system. Concern for the beef on dairy heifers arises because of increased variability in gain, cutability, and dressing percent in comparison to the steers. There is a need for using male sexed semen from the beef sires. Utilizing SimAngus bulls makes for a three-way cross, which will increase

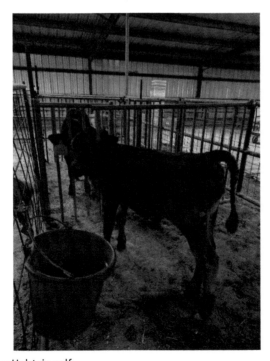

Fig. 7. SimAngus x Holstein calf.

heterosis and improve health of the resulting animal. The HOLSim program is backed by the IGS database, which includes nearly 20 million animals of various breeds and bred compositions, including dairy crosses.[9] The program keys in on the following variable among the bulls to choose from: (1) marbling, (2) ribeye, (3) size, and (4) calving ease. Using these parameters and querying the database revealed that SimAngus bulls made up nearly 81% of the bulls that met the criteria (with remainder compromising 3% Angus, 6% straight Continental bulls, and 10% other breed composites).

Simplot's program in Idaho has been in development for over 10 years (**Fig. 8** as an example of the Charolais cross color). The company saw a need for not only advantages in the end product but also production and efficiency in the feedlot. The animals in their feedlots needed to have growth and feed efficiency along with adequate muscling, that is, ribeye shape and size. Marbling has been consistent from the beef on dairy animals. Simplot continues to have in-house research done, including taste sensory, to create the best bulls to use on dairy cattle. They then take the data to their company-owned herd of Charolais. At this time, there are roughly 5000, 350 to 400 lb (136–181 kg) beef on dairy animals entering Simplot's feed yards per month.

Like Simplot, ABS Global (InFocus) recognized the need for specific beef sires to complement the dairy animal. The company saw that simply using beef EPDs and translating to the dairy cow did not always work. Therefore, they endeavored to create their own herd of cattle to meet the beef on dairy needs. They are targeting fertility, calving ease (low stillbirth %), feedlot performance, and finally carcass quality.

Other programs in the industry include Breeding to Feeding (LimFlex) at Alta, Genex, and Semex (**Fig. 9**) along with ProfitSource from Select Sires.

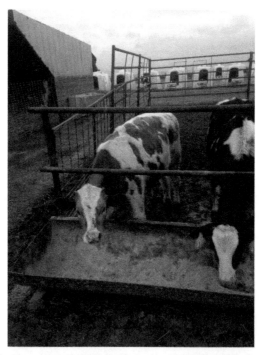

Fig. 8. Example of a Charolais x Holstein calf along a Holstein calf from a Midwest Dairy to show the color.

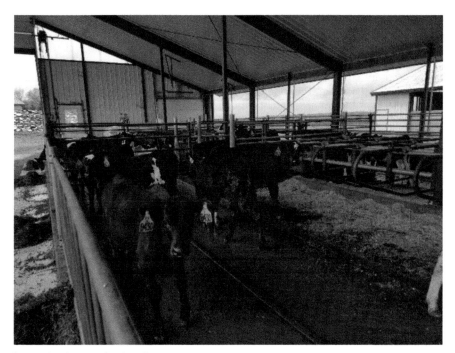

Fig. 9. LimFlex x Holstein calves.

Feeding Beef on Dairy Cattle

Although many areas of the country, that is, Desert Southwest, have successfully fed Holstein steers for decades, straight Holsteins tend to struggle in other parts of the country. Holsteins have thinner skin, less hair, and less backfat, which make them less able to handle colder climates. Beef on dairy crosses are better able to handle cold weather. Therefore, the industry is seeing more and more dairy beef crosses fed throughout the United States.

Typically, beef on dairy crosses are raised alongside Holsteins in calf ranches. They typically transition from the calf ranches or dairies to the feedyards at 175 to 200 kg. Because of this, the cattle are entering feedyards at a lighter weight than the yards are typically used to. One of the impacts of this is that turnover in the yard is reduced significantly, as the cattle will be on feed for over 300 days compared with yearling cattle that are normally on feed for half that period.

Owing to the long days on feed and tendency for dairy cattle to have digestive problems, more roughage is often fed to beef on dairy steers. Calves are typically grown on a higher roughage ration until they are 500 to 600 lb (225–275 kg), and then transitioned to finish ration until they reach harvest weight, typically 1360 lb (620 kg).

Gains on the beef on dairy cattle are better than straight Holsteins, but not quite as good as straight bred native beef cattle. However, because these cattle are generally started on feed at light weights, their conversions tend to be very desirable. Profitability on these cattle is driven to a large extent by the purchase price of the cattle. The premiums paid to the day-old calves tend to be high relative to Holstein calves, and these purchase prices are passed on to the feeder calf price entering the feedyard.

Growth-promoting technologies are prevalent across the industry and offer tremendous return on investment for dairy on beef animals. Cattle of dairy genetics are predisposed to bullying activity, and aggressive implants accentuate this behavior pattern. When bullying activity is observed, it is recommended to re-evaluate the implant program and possibly reduce the aggressiveness of the program to reduce bullying activity. Likewise, Ractopamine is commonly used throughout the industry. Unlike native beef, the dry matter intakes on these beef on dairy limit the amount of active ingredients consumed by the cattle.

In many areas of the country, cattle of dairy genetics are predisposed to a high incidence of liver abscesses. It was not unheard of to see 80% liver abscesses, with a majority of them being scored A+, or extreme. These A+ liver abscesses result in lower dressing percentage because of the trim associated with adherence of the abscess to the diaphragm or abdominal cavity. The cause of the high incidence of liver abscesses is not known, but is likely due to a combination of factors including roughage level, days on feed, and weather fluctuations. Unfortunately, anecdotal evidence suggests that the susceptibility of dairy beef cross cattle is closer to Holsteins than beef cattle. Feeding Tylan through the feeding period results in a dramatic reduction in liver abscesses.

DISCLOSURE

The authors have nothing to disclose.

REFERENCES

1. Berry DP, Amer PR, Evans RD, et al. A breeding index to rank beef bulls for use on dariy females to maximize profit. J Dairy Sci 2019;102:10056–72.
2. Eaglen SAE, Cole JB. What's going on with calving ease. Available at: https://www.naab-css.org/news/what-s-going-on-with-calving-ease. Accessed May 5, 2021.
3. Geiger C. Beef-on-dairy semen sales skyrocketed in 2018, . Hoard's dairyman. Available at: https://hoards.com/article-25428-beef-on-dairy-semen-sales-skyrocketed-in-2018.html. Accessed May 13, 2021.
4. Berry DP. Invited review: Beef-on-dairy——The generation of crossbred beef x dairy cattle. J Dairy Sci 2021;104:3789–819.
5. DelCurto T, Murphy T, and Moreaux S. Demographics and long-term outlook for western US beef sheep and horse industries and their importance for the forage industry. Proc. 2017 Western Alfalfa and Forage Symposium. Reno (NV). 2017; pp 87-99.
6. Berry DP, Ring SC. Short communication: Animal-level factors associated with whether a dairy female is mated to a dairy or beef bull. J Dairy Sci 2020;103: 8343–9.
7. Hanson M. Does breeding to beef sires alter dam productivity?. Available at: https://www.dairyherd.com/news/dairy-production/does-breeding-beef-sires-alter-dam-productivity. Accessed May 25, 2021.
8. Overton MW, Cabrera VE. Monitoring and quantifying the value of change in reproductive performance. In: Beede D, editor. Large dairy herd management. 3rd edition. Champaign (IL): American Dairy Science Association; 2017. p. 549–64.
9. Kemp C. Director American Simmental Association and IGS Commercial and Industry Operations. Personal communications. Accessed May 4, 2021.

10. Overton MW, Dhyvetter KC. Symposium review: An abundance of replacement heifers: What is the economic impact of raising more than are needed? J Dairy Sci 2020;103:3828–37.
11. Extension. Heifer Economics. Available at: https://dairy-cattle.extension.org/heifer-economics/. Accessed May 5, 2021.
12. DeVries A. Exploring the best combinations of genomics, semen type, and culling in dairy cattle. Available at: https://dairy-cattle.extension.org/exploring-the-best-combinations-of-genomics-semen-type-and-culling-in-dairy-cattle/. Accessed May 5, 2021.
13. Weigel M. Unlocking your heifer inventory goals. 2020. Available at: https://www.progressivedairy.com/topics/calves-heifers/unlocking-your-heifer-inventory-goals. Accessed May 5, 2021.
14. Halfman B, Sterry R. Dairy farm use, and criteria for use, of beef genetics on dairy females. 2019. Available at: https://fyi.extension.wisc.edu/wbic/files/2019/07/dairy-beef-survey-white-paper-Final-4-4-2019.pdf. Accessed May 13, 2021.
15. McWhorter T, Hutchinson JL, Norman HD, et al. Investigating conception rate for beef service sires bred to dairy cows and heifers. J Dairy Sci 2020;103:10374–82.
16. Coffeen P. Beef on dairy done right: How to make the crossbred calf the market desires. Available at: https://www.progressivedairy.com/topics/a-i-breeding/beef-on-dairy-done-right-how-to-make-the-crossbred-calf-the-market-desires. Accessed May 5, 2021.
17. Twomey AJ, Ring SC, McHugh N, et al. Carcass and efficiency metrics of beef cattle differ by whether the calf was born in a dairy or a beef herd. J Ani Sci 2020;98:skaa321.
18. Alberti PB, Panea B, Sanudo C, et al. Live weight, body size and carcass characteristics of young bulls of fifteen European breeds. Livest Sci 2008;114:19–30.

Acceptable Young Calf Vaccination Strategies— What, When, and How?

Christopher C.L. Chase, DVM, MS, PhD

KEYWORDS

- Bovine • Mucosal • Immunology • Vaccinology • Calves

KEY POINTS

- Management factors beginning with colostrum management for the calf are essential for good immune development and vaccine response.
- Vaccines are often viewed as a catch-all solution for management and nutrition errors; the "best" vaccine can never overcome these deficiencies.
- Calf vaccine protocols need to take into consideration animal flow, actual "disease" threats, and labor on the farm.

INTRODUCTION—IN THE BEGINNING, THERE WAS THE IMMUNE RESPONSE

The immune system consists of 3 lines of defense systems: mucosa epithelium, innate immunity, and adaptive or acquired immunity (**Fig. 1**) that work together to give cattle protection from disease. The mucosa epithelium of the respiratory and gastrointestinal (GI) system is the largest immune organ of the body and provides the barrier, "the kill zone" that eliminates 99.9% of all infections (**Fig. 2**).[1] The mucosa integrates all the components of the immune system: (1) barrier components (mucous and mucins, tight junctions); (2) innate immunity (macrophages, defensins, neutrophils, interferon, cytokines); and (3) adaptive immunity (secretory IgA and IgG, and T and B lymphocytes). This system is very susceptible to dehydration and changes in microbial populations. In addition, the mucosa epithelium, along with the lamina propria, is the immune "fire wall" (**Fig. 3**),[2] the regulatory system that provides "homeostasis" mechanisms that balance the immune system to provide a stable healthy internal environment to minimize inflammation (**Fig. 4**).[2] Homeostasis is dependent on both development of mucosal epithelium and the calf's microbiome. Once the mucosa epithelium is breached, the innate system is the first to be activated and responds almost immediately (**Fig. 5**). The adaptive response follows up 10 to 14 days later in naïve animals.

Department of Veterinary and Biomedical Sciences, South Dakota State University, PO Box 2175, SAR Room 119, N Campus Drive, Brookings, SD 57007, USA
E-mail address: Christopher.Chase@sdstate.edu

Vet Clin Food Anim 38 (2022) 17–37
https://doi.org/10.1016/j.cvfa.2021.11.002
vetfood.theclinics.com

Immune Responses

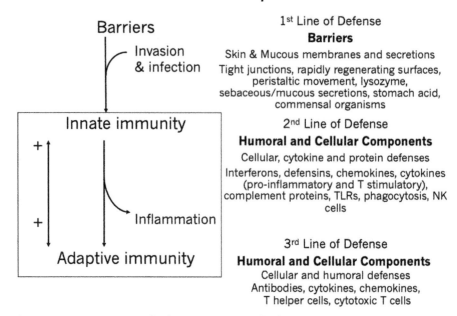

Barriers

Innate immunity

+ ↑

+

Inflammation

Adaptive immunity

Invasion & infection

1st Line of Defense

Barriers

Skin & Mucous membranes and secretions
Tight junctions, rapidly regenerating surfaces, peristaltic movement, lysozyme, sebaceous/mucous secretions, stomach acid, commensal organisms

2nd Line of Defense

Humoral and Cellular Components

Cellular, cytokine and protein defenses
Interferons, defensins, chemokines, cytokines (pro-inflammatory and T stimulatory), complement proteins, TLRs, phagocytosis, NK cells

3rd Line of Defense

Humoral and Cellular Components

Cellular and humoral defenses
Antibodies, cytokines, chemokines, T helper cells, cytotoxic T cells

Fig. 1. Immune responses: the barrier, innate, and adaptive immune components. (*From* Chase C. Neonatal Immune Development in the Calf and its Impact on the Vaccine response. *Veterinary Clinics of North America: Food Animal Practice.* Volume 24, Issue 1, March 2008, Pages 87-104.)

The immune system is regulated to prevent an over-response (too much of a good thing). The cumulative effect of these anti-inflammatory responses is to regulate the immune system, maintain homeostasis, and direct the immune response away from the memory response to the short-term antibody immune response. At the same time, overexpression of proinflammatory cytokines from infectious agents, feed intake issues (diet changes, fasting) and stress can result in immune dysfunction and an over-reactive immune system that can result in immunopathology and disease.[3,4]

THE GREAT UNKNOWN—PRENATAL DEVELOPMENT, FETAL IMPRINTING, COLOSTRUM DEVELOPMENT, AND THE CALF'S IMMUNE RESPONSE

The impact of nutrition and environmental exposure (weather, physical, microbial, etc.) to the pregnant cow on the developing fetal calf and its long-term health is a virtual unknown. The concept of fetal imprinting (aka epigenetic changes) has not been well studied in cattle.[5] Most studies in the pregnant dry cow have only looked at the effect of dry cow nutrition on colostrum and have failed to show measurable differences in colostral quality or absorption in the calf. In contrast, a few fetal imprinting studies in ruminants, where caloric restriction occurred during gestation, resulted in developmental changes in the enterocytes of the gut and the development of the gastrointestinal tract (GIT) of the calf.[6] Work at South Dakota State University in beef cows demonstrated that calves born from cows that received 80% of NRC

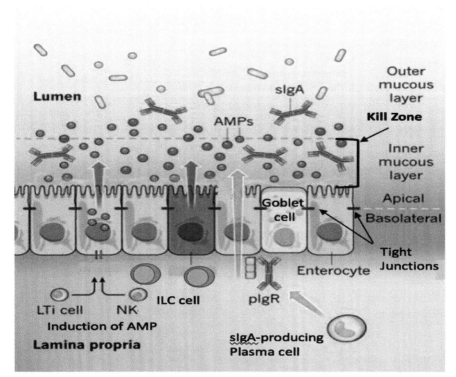

Fig. 2. The mucosal barrier. Mucosal epithelial cells (MEs) are integrated into a continuous, single-cell layer that is divided into apical and basolateral regions by tight junctions. MEs sense the microbiota and their metabolites to induce the production of antimicrobial peptides (AMPs). Goblet cells produce mucin and mucous, that is organized into a dense, more highly cross-linked inner proteoglycan gel that forms an adherent inner mucous layer, and a less densely cross-linked outer mucous layer. The outer layer is highly colonized by constituents of the microbiota. The inner mucous layer is largely impervious to bacterial colonization or penetration because of its high concentration of bactericidal AMPs, as well as commensals specific secretory IgA (sIgA), which is moved from their basolateral surface, where it is bound by the receptor, to the inner mucous layer. Responding to the microbiotal components, innate lymphoid cells (ILC), lymphoid tissue inducer cells (LTi), and natural killer cells (NK) produce cytokines, which stimulate AMP production and maintain the epithelial barrier. (*Adapted* from Maynard CL, Elson CO, Hatton RD, Weaver CT. Reciprocal interactions of the intestinal microbiota and immune system. *Nature.* 2012;489(7415):231-241. https://doi.org/10.1038/nature11551)

caloric intake over a 91-day period of midgestation had lower antibody responses at 4 months of age after weaning than calves born to cows receiving 100% NRC caloric requirement.[7] Microbial exposure during early human development primes fetal immune cells to be responsive to various antigens,[8] but these effects have not been measured in calves. The effect of excessive or deficiencies in vitamin and mineral levels on fetal calf development and subsequent health also has not been well characterized. This area of fetal programming and immune development will continue to be an area of great interest in understanding how to "maximize" calf health and well-being.

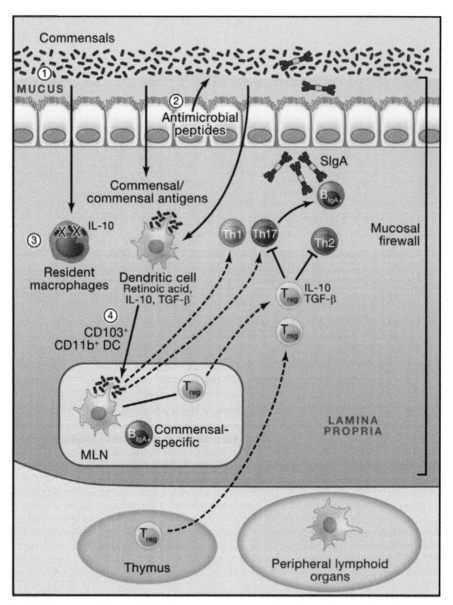

Fig. 3. The mucosal firewall. (1) The mucus represents the primary barrier limiting contact between the microbiota and host tissue preventing microbial translocation. (2) Epithelial cells produce antimicrobial peptides that also play a significant role in limiting exposure to the commensal microbiota. (3) Translocating commensals are rapidly eliminated by tissue-resident macrophages. (4) Commensals or commensal antigens can also be captured by DCs that traffic to the mesenteric lymph node from the lamina propria but do not penetrate further. Presentation of commensal antigens by these DCs leads to the differentiation of commensal-specific regulatory cells (T$_{reg}$), Th$_{17}$ cells, and IgA-producing B cells. Commensal-specific lymphocytes traffic to the lamina propria and Peyer's patches. In the Peyer's patches, T$_{reg}$ can further promote class switching and IgA generation against commensals. The combination of the epithelial barrier, mucus layer, IgA, and DCs and T cells comprises the "mucosal firewall," which limits the passage and exposure of commensals to the gut.

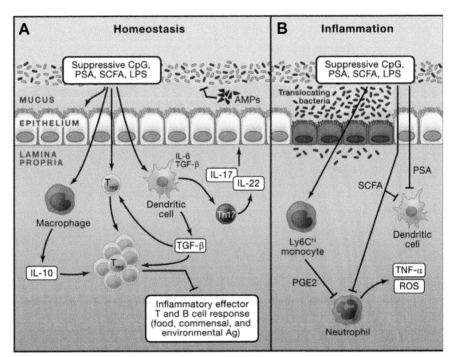

Fig. 4. (A) Commensals promote the induction of regulatory T cells via direct sensing of microbial products or metabolites by T cells or dendritic cells. Further commensals promote the induction of Th17 cells that can regulate the function and homeostasis of epithelial cells. In the context of inflammation, similar mechanisms may account for the regulatory role of the microbiota. (B) Commensal-derived metabolites can also have a local and systemic effect on inflammatory cells. For example, SCFA can inhibit neutrophil activation. Upon entrance into the tissue, inflammatory monocytes can also respond to microbial-derived ligands by producing mediators such as PGE$_2$ that limit neutrophil activation and tissue damage. (Belkaid Y, Hand TW. Role of the Microbiota in Immunity and Inflammation. *Cell*. 2014;157(1):121-141. https://doi.org/10.1016/j.cell.2014.03.011)

THE ESSENTIAL INGREDIENTS FOR A GOOD IMMUNE AND VACCINE RESPONSE— COLOSTRUM, HYDRATION, ENERGY, AND GOOD MANAGEMENT
Colostrum

Colostrum intake in the neonatal calf is essential because of its rich milieu of components for both physiologic and immunologic development—it provides important growth factors for GIT development, microbiome formation, and immune protection and development, to allow the newborn calf to establish homeostasis, which is essential for a protective response to vaccines (**Fig. 6**).[9] "Success" of colostrum management program has been measured based on total serum protein levels greater than 5.2 g/dL.[10] Dairy calves are at a distinct disadvantage, as their transition from colostrum to milk and milk to solid feed is much more abrupt than the "suckling calf" (**Fig. 7**)[11], which is not optimal for achieving "homeostasis" either at birth or weaning and for responding to vaccines. Colostrum is often primarily viewed as the "passive antibody" provider as its major contribution for calf health. Although maternal antibody is a major component, 3 other components have been underappreciated for their contribution to immune development and vaccine responses—vitamin A, microbiome/microbiome growth factors, and colostral cells.

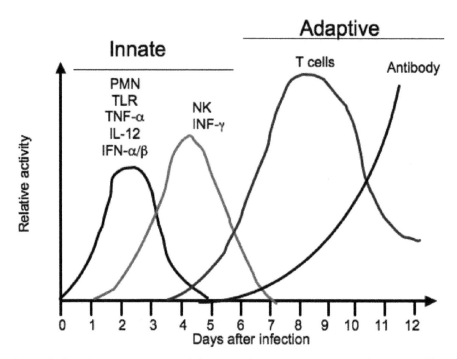

Fig. 5. The host immune response to infection and vaccines. PMN, neutrophils; TLR, toll-like receptor; TNF-α, tumor necrosis factor alpha-proinflammatory; IL-12, interleukin 12-proinflammatory; IFN-α/β, interferon alpha/beta; NK, natural killer cell; IFN-γ, interferon gamma-proinflammatory.

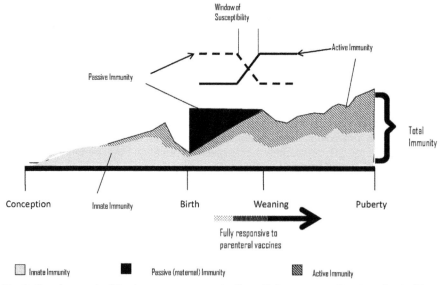

Fig. 6. Development of the immune response in the calf: from conception to puberty. (*From* Chase C. Neonatal Immune Development in the Calf and its Impact on the Vaccine response. *Veterinary Clinics of North America: Food Animal Practice.* Volume 24, Issue 1, March 2008, Pages 87-104.)

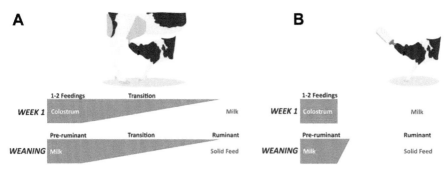

Fig. 7. Contrast in transition of colostrum and milk intakes in cow-calf suckling versus bottle suckling. (*A*) A calf suckling from the dam, as would occur in nature or in a beef cow-calf pair. During week 1, the calf would consume colostrum from the dam during the first 1 to 2 milkings, followed by transition milk in milkings 2 to 6 and mature milk by milkings 7 to 8. In nature, weaning would occur at approximately 8 months of life and would take place over 2 to 4 months. (*B*) A calf suckling a bottle, as occurs in commercial dairy production. On commercial dairy farms, calves are typically fed 1 or 2 meals of colostrum, followed by an abrupt transition to whole milk or milk replacer. Calves are typically weaned at 5 to 6 weeks of age to encourage early starter intake and rumen development. Weaning on commercial dairy farms is often abrupt and takes place over 1 to 2 weeks. (*Adapted from* Fischer, A.J., Villot, C., Niekerk, J.K. van, Yohe, T.T., Renaud, D.L., Steele, M.A., 2019. Nutritional regulation of gut function in dairy calves: From colostrum to weaning. Appl Animal Sci 35, 498–510. https://doi.org/10.15232/aas.2019-01887.)

Vitamin A

Calves are born vitamin A deficient, and colostrum is rich in vitamin A and its active metabolic forms (retinol, retinal, retinoic acid, and provitamin β-carotene).[12] These metabolites, which are essential for mucosal immune and vaccine responses in the neonatal (**Fig. 8**),[13] are not present in injectable vitamin A products. Calves with

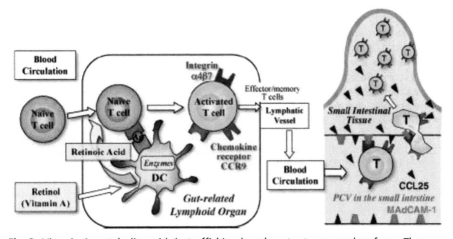

Fig. 8. Vitamin A metabolites aids in trafficking lymphocytes to mucosal surfaces. There are fewer T and B cells seen in mucosal lymphoid follicles with vitamin A deficiency. (*Adapted from* Iwata, M., 2009. Retinoic acid production by intestinal dendritic cells and its role in T-cell trafficking. Semin Immunol 21, 8–13. https://doi.org/10.1016/j.smim.2008.09.002.)

vitamin A deficiency respond poorly to nasal vaccines and are more susceptible to bovine respiratory syncytial virus (BRSV) infections.[14] Neonatal calves with vitamin A deficiency were 2.8 times more likely to die.[15]

Microbiome/microbiome growth factors

A key feature in the development of an immune response is a highly diverse microbiome in the gut. This development requires 3 components: microbiome organisms, microbiome growth factors, and mucosal cell growth factors.[16] Colostrum accelerates GIT microbiome development.[11] Animals fed colostrum within 12 hours of birth, have 2 to 4 logs more of commensal organisms than calves not fed colostrum, and the quantity of beneficial bacteria was higher, while the colonization of *Escherichia coli* was reduced (**Fig. 9**).[16] Interestingly, pasteurization of colostrum increased the levels of colostral microbiome growth factors (oligosaccharides) and the proportion of beneficial GIT in the lower small intestinal tract,[16,17] in addition to reducing coliform bacteria and *Mycobacterium* associated with Johne disease.[11] Oligosaccharides have also been associated with enhanced IgG absorption from colostrum. Mucosal growth factors like insulin-like growth factor 1 (IGF-1) and glucagon-like peptide-1 and -2 enhance GIT growth and microbiome development.[11]

Colostral cells

The feeding of colostrum containing live colostral cells results in higher numbers of activated T helper cells, less respiratory disease,[18] and higher vaccine responses, including higher B cell numbers in calves vaccinated between 1 and 4 months of age.[19] Pasteurization or freezing mitigates the positive effect of the live cells, making colostrum management an important factor, depending on the type of disease burden at the farm, especially for the prevention of Johne disease.

Hydration and Nutrition

One of the most critical issues in poor responses to vaccines is when animals are dehydrated and/or energy "starved." The immune system requires hydration and energy for the barrier to be effective and for the immune system to actively respond and develop an effective and long-lasting immune response. Hydration in the young calf has been underappreciated. Dairy calves, given free access to water from birth, consumed more milk, grew better, and weighed more than calves given free access to water at 17 days of age.[20] This effect on growth was seen out to 5 months of age, when the study was ended. Although not statistically significant, the acute-phase protein, haptoglobin (HPG), an innate protein induced by inflammation, was twice as high at 14 days of age in the calves not receiving free access to water as compared with the calves receiving free-choice water from birth.[20] Another large calf study measured calf outcomes based on a single HPG test at 8 days of age. The average HPG from 1365 calves from 15 farms was at levels similar to the levels seen in the calves not receiving free-choice water in the Wickramasinghe study.[21] Calves with higher HPG levels at 8 days of age had higher disease and higher mortality.[21] This implies that the lower HPG levels seen with calves receiving free-choice water from birth have long-term health consequences, which should include better vaccine responses. The immune system is a major consumer of energy and in times of negative energy, like seen in the newborn calf and newly weaned calf, can be difficult times for the immune system to respond. The immune response requires energy, protein, vitamins, and trace minerals. Both malnutrition and overfeeding may result in impairment of immune function and increased susceptibility to disease, because of a deficiency or excess of proteins or calories, or a relative imbalance in vitamin or trace

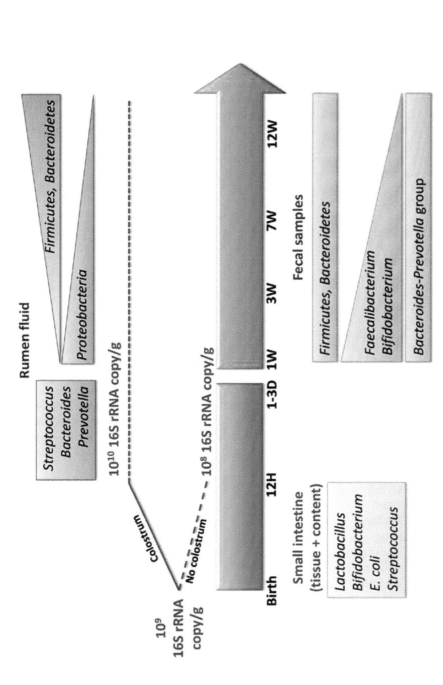

Fig. 9. Colonization of neonatal calf rumen/gut, immediately postpartum and within the first 12 weeks of life. (*Adapted from* Malmuthuge N, Griebel PJ, Guan LL. The Gut Microbiome and Its Potential Role in the Development and Function of Newborn Calf Gastrointestinal Tract. Frontiers Vet Sci 2015;2:36. https://doi.org/10.3389/fvets.2015.00036.)

mineral content.[22] As calves are born with only 3% to 4% of body weight as fat, they can become emaciated and die if energy balance is negative for more than 3 to 5 days.[23] The use of milk replacers and calf starters, supplemented with higher levels of butyric and linolenic acids, reduced the proinflammatory response, increased the anti-inflammatory responses after vaccination and increased antibody responses.[24] It also decreased diarrhea, *Clostridial*-associated disease, and improved average daily gain and feed efficiency.[24] Animals under intensive production conditions typically have a completely controlled diet. It is very important that the diet, especially the vitamin and trace mineral content, be optimally formulated. Key vitamins and minerals for optimal immune function include vitamins A, C, E, and the B complex vitamins, copper (Cu), zinc (Zn), magnesium (Mg), manganese (Mn), iron (Fe), and selenium (Se). Of these, zinc, copper, and selenium are the "immune microminerals." The balance of these constituents is especially important as excess or deficiency in one component may influence the availability or requirement for another. Zinc is involved in protein synthesis and antibody formation, cell differentiation, and enzyme formation and function. Zinc also plays a major role in skin and mucosal integrity, the first line of defense of the immune system. It is also essential for innate immune responses.[25] Copper and manganese are directly involved with cell-mediated immunity and protein matrix formation during the healing process. Copper has been linked with the ability of isolated neutrophils to kill yeast and bacterial infections. Selenium is an essential antioxidant.[26] Manganese plays a role in facilitating the "germ-killing" function of macrophages.[27]

MANAGEMENT AND BIOSECURITY

Many stressors cause major dysfunction to the immune system and affect vaccine responses. Disease can be managed by the diligence of the producer (**Fig. 10**). These animal husbandry practices are necessary, and their deficiencies cannot be "corrected" by vaccines (see **Fig. 10**). The nutritional aspects have been discussed earlier. Housing, particularly heat abatement, airflow and proper "winter" environment are critical. An often-overlooked issue in group housing with automatic calf feeders,

- **Good Husbandry**
  - **Nutrition**
    - Feed
    - Water
  - **Housing**
    - Ventilation
    - Heating/Cooling
    - Electrical issues
  - **Managing Procedures**
    - Surgical Procedures
    - Vaccination
    - Transportation
    - Handling
- **Biosecurity**

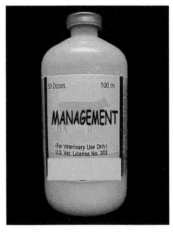

Fig. 10. Management factors to improve health and immune response.

waterers and/or lockups can be low-level electrical forces. Common procedures such as dehorning (disbudding), castration, and vaccination that are often done concurrently, need to be implemented carefully particularly in areas of pain management for surgical procedures and "immune reactions" that occur after "normal vaccination" such as inappetence, listlessness, and febrile response. With the increased use of off-site calf rearing facilities, transportation and handling also need to be managed carefully. Finally, biosecurity procedures cannot be neglected. This begins with testing of neonatal calves for bovine viral diarrhea virus (BVDV) persistent infection (PI). Proper cleaning and disinfection procedures of housing, transportation (trucks and trailers), surgical instruments, and milk feeding equipment, along with proper use of personal protective equipment (boots, gloves, etc.) are essential. Traffic flow and signage also need to be implemented. Single use of hypodermic needles is also essential.

DO I REALLY NEED TO VACCINATE THE YOUNG CALF? YES, BUT PROBABLY LATER THAN WE THINK

In assessing vaccine protocols, it has been my experience that calves are vaccinated too soon and too often. Simplifying protocols frequently can result in reduced morbidity, reduced expense, and improved gain. The use of parenteral 5-way viral vaccines in dairy calves at 2 and 5 weeks of age (particularly if given at 2 weeks of age) has actually resulted in slightly higher morbidity and mortality and no difference in performance.[28] Interestingly, only higher maternal antibody titers to BRSV and bovine herpesvirus 1 (BHV-1) in the calf have been associated with less bovine respiratory disease (BRD) in either vaccinated or nonvaccinated calves.[29] Higher titers to BVDV, bovine coronavirus, or *Mannheimia haemolytica* were not associated with reduced BRD.

The newborn calf is immunologically naïve at birth. It has had no chance to enhance adaptive immunity by "experience" because of the protective environment in the uterus. It is further handicapped by maternal factors and the hormonal influences of parturition, and by its lack of antibodies in circulation and in the tissues. The ingestion of colostrum is essential for providing the neonate with immunologic protection during at least the first 2 to 4 weeks of life. Although all the essential immune components are present in the neonate at birth, many of the components are not functional until the calf is at least 3 weeks of age and may continue to develop until puberty (see **Fig. 6**).[9] This ongoing maturity of the immune system in the developing neonate, coupled with maternal antibody interference, makes vaccination strategy more complex. The mucosa epithelium provides immune function very early, making most intranasal and oral vaccines effective in calves less than a week of age. Parenterally administered modified live virus (MLV) vaccine responses begin at 7 to 10 days after birth, although BVDV MLV vaccines should be avoided. particularly in dairy calves before at least 2 months of age, as the major BVDV vaccine strains inhibit innate immune bacterial killing for 10 to 14 days after vaccination.[30] The use of oral coronavirus/rotavirus vaccines in the neonatal is not an effective strategy to prevent these diarrheal diseases, as colostral antibodies neutralize the vaccine virus.[31,32] Bacterial parenteral vaccines typically do not have much response in animals less than 3 weeks of age, with the exception of *Clostridium perfringens* toxoids that have an immune response when administered at 3 days of age.[33]

WHAT? PATHOGENS/IMMUNOGENS AND TYPES OF VACCINES
What to Vaccinate for? What Pathogens Make Sense?

Calf vaccine programs are probably the most effective against viral pathogens (BHV-1 [IBR], BRSV, and BVDV). This is because many of the cattle bacterial pathogens

(*Histophilus somni*, *M haemolytica*, *Pasteurella multocida*, *Moraxella spp.*, *Mycoplasma bovis*, *Salmonella typhimurium*, and *C perfringens*) are "normal inhabitants" of the bovine microbiome and they are "endemic" in most herds.[16,34] Stressors that were discussed earlier play a major role in allowing these "normal" bugs to become pathogenic. Looking at a herd, it is essential to have a strong diagnostic program in place to get accurate pathogen diagnosis. With next-generation sequencing, diagnostic PCR, and good old-fashioned pathology and microbiology isolation, there has never been a better time to determine which pathogens are occurring and when. Being strategic in vaccination requires targeting those pathogens on that farm or ranch. A term that we have learned from COVID-19 is Replication Rate called R "naught" (R_0).[35,36] Replication rate is the number of susceptible animals that one infected animal can infect (**Fig. 11**). Probably, one of the most "infectious" viruses is BRSV (**Table 1**). BRSV has been estimated to have an $R_0 \sim 36$. A BRSV susceptible animal (neonate) is highly susceptible to BRSV infection because of the high R_0. In a herd with BRSV disease history, BRSV vaccination would be on the top of the list. Once an animal is infected with BRSV and endemic in the herd, the immunity is not perfect but R_0 is 1.1 so BRSV is barely circulating in the herd (see **Table 1**). For IBR and BVDV transient infections, the rate is around ~ 3—meaning one infected animal

Basic reproduction number

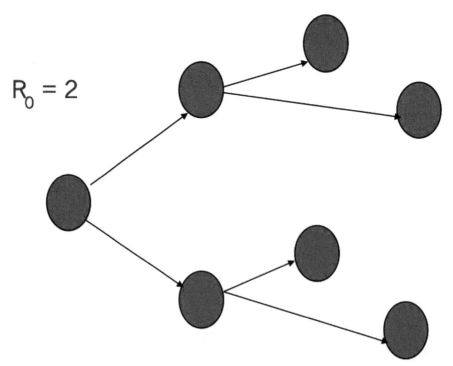

$R_0 = 2$

Fig. 11. The basic reproduction number (R naught). In this example, the $R_0 = 2$, meaning that one infected animal can infect 2 susceptible animals.

Table 1
Herd immunity thresholds for selected bovine vaccine-preventable diseases

Disease	R_o	Herd Immunity Needed to Prevent
BVDV PI	∞ [d]	>95%
BRSV-naive	36.5[a]	>95%
BHV-1-naive	3.2[b,e]	75%–86%
BVDV-transient	0.25[d]–3.4[c]	70%–80%
BRSV-endemic	1.14[a]	50%–60%
BHV-1-latency	0.5[e]	0%
COVID19	2–3	60%–66%

[a] M.C.M. de Jong, et al. Am. J. Vet. Res. 1996;57, 628-633.
[b] Bosch, J.C., et al. Vaccine. 1998;16, 265–271.
[c] Moerman, A., et al. Veterinary Record. 1993;132, 622-626.
[d] Sarrazin, S., et al. The Veterinary Journal 202, 244-249.
[e] Brock, J., et al. Vet Res. 2020;51, 124.

shedding virus could potentially infect 3 susceptible animals (see **Table 1**). By the time we get 70% to 80% of the animals either infected or protected from vaccination, the occurrence of infections to those viruses will be low and herd immunity has been achieved (see **Table 1**). The BVDV PI animal is the one case that totally destroys the concept of herd immunity. As the BVDV PI animal continually sheds virus, any susceptible animal is at risk of infection. This makes the R_0 for a herd with BVDV PI of ∞ "infinity" indicating that a herd with a PI animal can never vaccinate its way out of the threat of BVDV. Endemic viral infections frequently include rotavirus and bovine coronavirus, along with *C perfringens,* which represent a threat to the newborn susceptible animals. Environmental pathogens like *Bacillus anthracis* (anthrax), *Leptospira* spp., *E coli, Campylobacter* require considerations based on herd history and locality. Finally, Brucella abortus represents a "regulatory" vaccine.

HOW DO WE VACCINATE—ROUTE?
Mucosal Delivery Versus Parenteral Delivery

Mucosal delivery of vaccine either orally or intranasal is a strategy that has been used for 3 reasons: (1) mucosal responses occur earlier in the neonatal calf than parenteral, (2) the presence of systemic maternal antibody has little effect on generating antigenic mass necessary for developing an immune response that occurs after immunizing with a mucosal vaccine (in the face of maternal antibody [IFOMA]), and (3) mucosal vaccination results in the generation of secretory IgA that is produced locally and protects mucosal surfaces where most pathogens are colonized and/or infect the host (**Fig. 12**). For all vaccines, mucosal or parenteral, the critical immune reactions occur in the draining lymph node (see **Fig. 12**; **Fig. 13**). With the right adjuvanted parenteral MLV vaccine, a protective mucosal IgA response can occur IFOMA.[37] The paradigm that only mucosal vaccines result in the immune response IFOMA and induce mucosal IgA is not true. The key ingredient for a parenteral MLV vaccine to induce mucosal immunity is the adjuvant. Most adjuvants cannot overcome IFOMA and/or produce a mucosal IgA response (see **Fig. 13**). The more sophisticated oil-saponin adjuvants have this ability.[37]

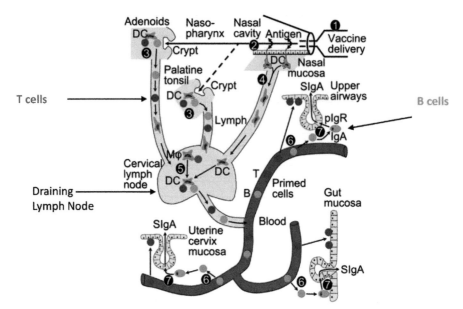

Fig. 12. Where does the immune response occur with mucosal vaccine? (1) Delivery of nasal vaccine; (2) uptake of vaccine antigen through nasal mucosa; (3) immune induction in nasal-associated lymphoid tissue (NALT), including tonsils; (4) antigen targeting and migration of mucosal dendritic cells (DCs) to regional draining lymph node; (5) immune induction and amplification in regional (cervical) lymph nodes by antigen-loaded DCs and macrophages (MΦ); (6) compartmentalized homing and exit of NALT-induced T and B cells to secretory effector sites in airways, gut, and uterine cervix; and (7) local production and polymeric Ig receptor (pIgR)-mediated external transport of dimeric IgA to generate secretory IgA (SIgA). (*Adapted from* Brandtzaeg P. Potential of nasopharynx-associated lymphoid tissue for vaccine responses in the airways. Am J Respir Crit Care Med 2011;183:1595–1604.)

Needleless Injections

Needle-free injection devices (NFIDs) result in a high-pressure stream that penetrates the epidermis and dermis with some subcutaneous penetration.[38] NFID-administered vaccines can use half to a tenth of the dose required for intramuscular vaccines because of the higher antigen dispersion and contact with the antigen-presenting cells found in the skin. The use of NFID decreases the number of needle-stick injuries. Needle-free devices also have disadvantages, including start-up cost of the equipment, exhaustible gas-storage infrastructure (for those systems using compressed or $CO2$ gas system), technical and operational expertise (training of the operators and maintenance of the units), and inability to completely replace needle-syringe devices. The cost of the equipment varies depending on the type of needle-free injector and there are additional associated costs with maintenance and infrastructure, especially with compressed gas devices. The needle-free application requires a consistent application method. Needle-free devices are calibrated to deliver the vaccine when the needle-free device is perpendicular (90°) to the skin. Vaccinations made at more acute or oblique angles will affect the distribution of the vaccine in the tissue. In addition, because of the moving parts and gas system, regular maintenance is required. Finally, there is no "one-size-fits-all" needle-free device for all applications that require injections. Humidity, cattle breed, hide condition (hair coat, mud, snow, etc.), and age

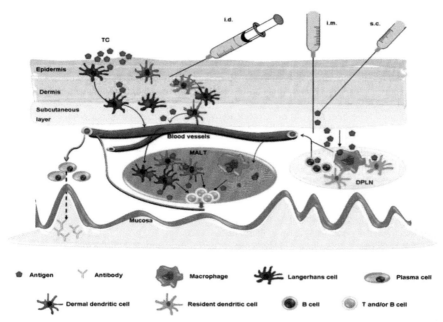

Fig. 13. Properly adjuvanted parenteral vaccines can induce mucosal IgA responses via the draining lymph node. DPLN, draining peripheral lymph node; MALT, mucosal-associated lymph tissue. (*From* Su F, Patel GB, Hu S, et al. Induction of mucosal immunity through systemic immunization: Phantom or reality? Hum Vaccin Immunother 2016;12:1070–1079.)

of the animal affect the elasticity and thickness of the hide, greatly changing the force required for correct delivery. Different ages, breeds of cattle, treatment dose, and viscosity of injection substance require different injection volume, injection pressure, and even different NFIDs. Adoption of needle-free devices in the US cattle industry has been slow, although there has been better adaption in the swine industry, driven by foreign markets that require the use of NFID. Reasons for this low industry implementation rate involve cost of the unit and associated maintenance and infrastructure costs, higher complexity than needle-syringe device, availability of devices (a smaller handheld injector that is used in Europe is not available in the United States), uncertainty if the animal was vaccinated (ie, no physical sensation that the animal was vaccinated and/or a "wet" appearance at the injection site), and requirement for training.

MLV and inactivated—together is even better

MLV vaccines have been used because of the good antibody response, longer duration of immunity, fewer doses needed per animal, and lower cost. To a lesser extent, modified live bacterial vaccines have also been used (*Brucella abortus, M haemolytica, Pasteurella multocida*, and *Salmonella dublin*). These MLV vaccines are administered intramuscularly, intranasally, or subcutaneously. As the basis for establishing a good immune response, they are optimal. Although the return to virulence in MLV vaccines has been minimal, mutations will occur and there is some risk of new strains arising. Nonadjuvanted MLV vaccines also fail to booster well-vaccinated animals. Active vaccine immunity neutralizes vaccine virus preventing the MLV from replicating and preventing a booster immune response.[39,40] Unlike maternal interference, this active immune interference never goes away in well-vaccinated animals. The animal's

---

Box 1
Vaccine schedule

Neonatal Calves
Respiratory Diseases
MLV intranasal vaccines (depends on maternal antibody levels—many MLV IM or SC *not effective before 30–45 days*—only adjuvanted MLV IM or SC *likely effective before 30-45 days*)
Branding time-beef MLV IM or SC, MLV adjuvanted, not affected by maternal antibody; inactivated viral vaccines??
Enteric Diseases
Rota-coronavirus MLV-1 dose—within the first week of life—not recommended because of maternal interference and later onset of protection.
Clostridial perfringens Toxoid in the first 3 to 5 days after birth

Calves (>3 months)
2 to 3 weeks before weaning
MLV-1 dose (BVDV 1 & 2, BRSV, BHV-1, PI-3)
Inactivated-2 doses (BVDV 1 & 2, BRSV, BHV-1, PI-3)
Bacterial respiratory disease? (*M haemolytica, H somni*, and/or *P multocida*)
Clostridial diseases
At weaning
MLV-immune dysfunction—delay—a few days to a month
Inactivated-2 doses
Bacterial respiratory disease?
Clostridial diseases
2 to 3 weeks after weaning
MLV-1 dose
Inactivated-2 doses
Bacterial respiratory disease?
Clostridial diseases

Heifer Development
Respiratory and Reproductive Diseases
Heifers (prebreeding)—Heifers need to receive at least 1 dose of MLV before addition to the breeding herd (1 dose should contain BVDV Singer strain)
MLV-2 doses—BVDV and BHV-1
  more than 6 and 2 months before breeding
Inactivated viral-2 doses
  5 and 2 weeks before breeding
Leptospirosis-2 doses
  5 and 2 weeks before breeding
Brucellosis-1 dose

---

immune system cannot differentiate between a natural infection or vaccine virus. Another issue with MLV IBR (BHV-1) vaccines is that they result in latency and their continued use throughout the life of the animal will ensure that BHV-1 will be present in the herd, even though the rates of the shed are between 0.13% and 2.6% of the animals' shed.[36]

Inactivated vaccines contain chemically or physically treated bacteria, toxins, and/or viruses. There is no danger of replication in the vaccinated animal of the pathogen or adventitious agents that may be present in an MLV. Improved adjuvants have increased the scope and duration of inactivated virus immunity. They have several disadvantages including cost, and more doses required per animal. Inactivated vaccines generate cell-mediated responses.[41,42] Interestingly, there is ample evidence that inactivated vaccines can effectively boost MLV vaccines.[40,43–46] Inactivated vaccines have also been shown to decrease BHV-1 latency shed rates.[44]

Frequency of vaccination. No more than 1 to 2 doses of MLV or 2 to 3 doses of inactivated vaccines should be administered in young calves less than 4 months of age to develop good herd immunity against respiratory diseases (**Box 1**).

Interval between doses of vaccine. In all animals, after vaccination, there is expansion in the populations of responding T-cells and B-cells. To have a complete and mature immune response, this T-cell and B-cell expansion must not only stop, but an active process of cell death (apoptosis) must also occur. This "waning process" allows "culling" T-cells or B-cells that may be poor responders or even cause autoimmunity to be removed by apoptosis. This whole process from vaccination to achieving mature immune response homeostasis takes at least 3 weeks (**Fig. 14**). This fully developed mature primary response can then be boosted to get a true anamnestic secondary response. In many cases, cattle vaccine primary and booster doses are administered at 2-week intervals. In young calves, this is done to provide an opportunity to make sure that the calves develop a primary response in the face of maternal immunity. The adjuvants that are used with most commercial vaccines provide superior immune development over older generation adjuvants like alum. In most instances, if primary vaccination occurs after 3 weeks of age, booster vaccination beyond 3 weeks and even longer will be efficacious (see **Fig. 14**). The dogma that revaccination must occur within 2 weeks of the primary vaccination is not true and the anamnestic response will be better if we wait longer.

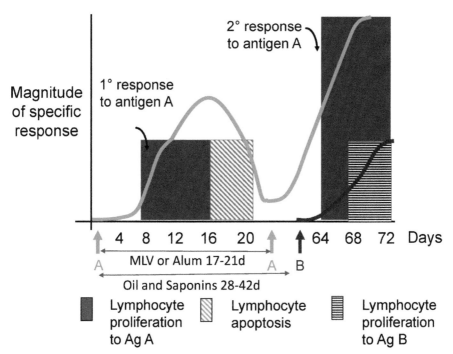

Fig. 14. Importance of timing and the booster response is dependent on the type of vaccine and/or adjuvant.

SUMMARY

Management of the calf's immune system is not a simple process. Stressors and nutrition often compromise immunity. It is important that vaccinations be given at optimal times and that vaccination is not overused. Vaccination can never overcome poor management.

DISCLOSURE

Dr C.C.L. Chase has received research funding and/or compensation for continuing education speaking events from Arm & Hammer Animal Health, Bayer Animal Health, Boehringer Ingelheim Animal Health, Diamond V Animal Health, Elanco Animal Health, Hipra, Lallemand Animal Health, Novartis Animal Health, Merial Animal Health, Merck Animal Health, Zinpro, and Zoetis Animal Health.
(Belkaid Y, Hand TW. Role of the Microbiota in Immunity and Inflammation. *Cell.* 2014;157(1):121-141. https://doi.org/10.1016/j.cell.2014.03.011)

REFERENCES

1. Maynard CL, Elson CO, Hatton RD, et al. Reciprocal interactions of the intestinal microbiota and immune system. Nature 2012;489(7415):231–41.
2. Belkaid Y, Hand TW. Role of the Microbiota in Immunity and Inflammation. Cell 2014;157(1):121–41.
3. Bradford BJ, Swartz TH. Review: Following the smoke signals: inflammatory signaling in metabolic homeostasis and homeorhesis in dairy cattle. Animal 2020;14:s144–54.
4. McGill JL, Sacco RE. The Immunology of Bovine Respiratory Disease. Vet Clin North Am Food Anim Pract 2020;36:333–48.
5. O'Doherty AM, MacHugh DE, Spillane C, et al. Genomic imprinting effects on complex traits in domesticated animal species. Front Genet 2015;6:156.
6. Steele MA, Malmuthuge N, Guan LL. Dietary Factors Influencing the Development of the Ruminant Gastrointestinal Tract. Semantic Scholar 2015. Available at. https://www.semanticscholar.org/paper/Dietary-Factors-Influencing-the-Development-of-the-Steele-Malmuthuge/be93a3cae9260236d4f45af295cd23f2d51-6bc2b. July 25, 2021.
7. Taylor A. The Effects of Maternal Energy Restriction During Mid-Gestation on Growth Performance, Immune Function, and Gene Expression in the Resultant Beef Offspring. PhD Dissertation 2014, South Dakota State University. Available at: https://openprairie.sdstate.edu/cgi/viewcontent.cgi?article=2598&context=-etd. July 25, 2021.
8. Mishra A, Lai GC, Yao LJ, et al. Microbial exposure during early human development primes fetal immune cells. Cell 2021;184:3394–409.e20.
9. Chase C, Hurley DJ, Reber AJ. Neonatal Immune Development in the Calf and Its Impact on Vaccine Response. Vet Clin North Am Food Anim Pract 2008;24:87–104.
10. Atkinson DJ, von Keyserlingk MAG, Weary DM. Benchmarking passive transfer of immunity and growth in dairy calves. J Dairy Sci 2017;100:3773–82.
11. Fischer AJ, Villot C, van Niekerk JK, et al. Invited Review: Nutritional regulation of gut function in dairy calves: From colostrum to weaning. Appl Anim Sci 2019;35:498–510.
12. McGrath BA, Fox PF, McSweeny PLH, et al. Composition and properties of bovine colostrum: a review. Dairy Sci Tech 2016;96:133–58.

13. Iwata M. Retinoic acid production by intestinal dendritic cells and its role in T-cell trafficking. Semin Immunol 2009;21:8–13.
14. McGill JL, Kelly SM, Guerra-Maupome M, et al. Vitamin A deficiency impairs the immune response to intranasal vaccination and RSV infection in neonatal calves. Sci Rep 2019;9:15157.
15. Waldner CL, Uehlinger FD. Factors associated with serum vitamin A and vitamin E concentrations in beef calves from Alberta and Saskatchewan and the relationship between vitamin concentrations and calf health outcomes. Can J Anim Sci 2017;97:65–82.
16. Malmuthuge N, Griebel PJ, Guan LL. The Gut Microbiome and Its Potential Role in the Development and Function of Newborn Calf Gastrointestinal Tract. Front Vet Sci 2015;2:36.
17. Fischer AJ, Malmuthuge N, Guan LL, et al. Short communication: The effect of heat treatment of bovine colostrum on the concentration of oligosaccharides in colostrum and in the intestine of neonatal male Holstein calves. J Dairy Sci 2018;101:401–7.
18. Langel SN, Wark WA, Garst SN, et al. Effect of feeding whole compared with cell-free colostrum on calf immune status: The neonatal period. J Dairy Sci 2015;98:3729–40.
19. Langel SN, Wark WA, Garst SN, et al. Effect of feeding whole compared with cell-free colostrum on calf immune status: Vaccination response. J Dairy Sci 2016;99:3979–94.
20. Wickramasinghe HKJP, Kramer AJ, Appuhamy JADRN. Drinking water intake of newborn dairy calves and its effects on feed intake, growth performance, health status, and nutrient digestibility. J Dairy Sci 2019;102:377–87.
21. Murray CF, Windeyer MC, Duffield TF, et al. Associations of serum haptoglobin in newborn dairy calves with health, growth, and mortality up to 4 months of age. J Dairy Sci 2014;97:7844–55.
22. Godden SM, Lombard JE, Woolums AR. Colostrum Management for Dairy Calves. Vet Clin North Am Food Anim Pract 2019;35:535–56.
23. Sockett D, Behr M, Earlywine T. Low Temperatures and Negative Energy Balance in Calves. Wisconsin Veterinary Diagnostic Laboratory Website, posted January 9, 2014. 2014. Available at: https://www.wvdl.wisc.edu/index.php/important-notice-pertaining-low-temperatures-negative-energy-balance-calves/. July 24, 2021.
24. Hill TM, VandeHaar MJ, Sordillo LM, et al. Fatty acid intake alters growth and immunity in milk-fed calves. J Dairy Sci 2011;94:3936–48.
25. Bonaventura P, Benedetti G, Albarède F, et al. Zinc and its role in immunity and inflammation. Autoimmun Rev 2015;14(4):277–85.
26. Sordillo LM. Selenium-dependent regulation of oxidative stress and immunity in periparturient dairy cattle. Vet Med Int 2013;4:154045–8.
27. Sordillo LM. Nutritional strategies to optimize dairy cattle immunity. J Dairy Sci 2016;99(6):4967–82.
28. Windeyer MC, Leslie KE, Godden SM, et al. The effects of viral vaccination of dairy heifer calves on the incidence of respiratory disease, mortality, and growth. J Dairy Sci 2012;95:6731–9.
29. Windeyer MC, Leslie KE, Godden SM, et al. Association of bovine respiratory disease or vaccination with serologic response in dairy heifer calves up to three months of age. Am J Vet Res 2015;76:239–45.

30. Roth JA, Kaeberle ML. Suppression of neutrophil and lymphocyte function induced by a vaccinal strain of bovine viral diarrhea virus with and without the administration of ACTH. Am J Vet Res 1983;44:2366–72.
31. Bonnema J. In Vitro Neutralization of Calf-Guard® with Colostral Whey: Using Lab Results to Understand the Outcome at the Calf-Level. 2018. Available at: https://firstdefensecalfhealth.com/wp-content/uploads/2020/08/In_Vitro_Neutralization_of_Calf-Guard.pdf. July 25, 2021.
32. Zaane DV, Ijzerman J, Leeuw PWD. Intestinal antibody response after vaccination and infection with rotavirus of calves fed colostrum with or without rotavirus antibody. Vet Immunol Immunopathol 1986;11:45–63.
33. Fleenor WA, Stott GH. Quantification of bovine IgG, IgM and IgA antibodies to Clostridium perfringens B-toxin by enzyme immunoassay. II. Systemic effects of maternally derived antibodies on immunization of newborn calves. Vet Immunol Immunopathol 1983;4:633–54.
34. Osman R, Malmuthuge N, González-Cano P, et al. Development and Function of the Mucosal Immune System in the Upper Respiratory Tract of Neonatal Calves. Annu Rev Anim Biosci 2018;6:141–55.
35. Greenhalgh D, Diekmann O, de Jong MCM. Subcritical endemic steady states in mathematical models for animal infections with incomplete immunity. Math Biosci 2000;165:1–25.
36. Koeijer A A de, Diekmann O, Jong MC M de. Calculating the time to extinction of a reactivating virus, in particular bovine herpes virus. Math Biosci 2008;212:111–31.
37. Kolb EA, Buterbaugh RE, Rinehart CL, et al. Protection against bovine respiratory syncytial virus in calves vaccinated with adjuvanted modified live vaccine administered in the face of maternal antibody. Vaccine 2020;38:298–308.
38. Chase C. What's the future in transdermal devices in swine? National Hog Farmer (NHF) Health and Welfare column. June 20, 2017. Available at: http://www.nationalhogfarmer.com/animal-health/what-s-future-transdermal-devices-swine. July 25, 2021.
39. Fulton RW, Confer AW, Burge LJ, et al. Antibody responses by cattle after vaccination with commercial viral vaccines containing bovine herpesvirus-1, bovine viral diarrhea virus, parainfluenza-3 virus, and bovine respiratory syncytial virus immunogens and subsequent revaccination at day 140. Vaccine 1995;13(8):725–33.
40. Royan G. Comparison of the BVDV, BHV-1, and BRSV Anamnestic Response to Modified-live or Inactivated Vaccines in Calves Previously Vaccinated with a Modified-live Virus Vaccine. Bov Pract 2009;43(1):44–50.
41. Sandbulte MR, Roth JA. Priming of multiple T cell subsets by modified-live and inactivated bovine respiratory syncytial virus vaccines. Vet Immunol Immunopathol 2003;95(3–4):123–33.
42. Stevens ET, Zimmerman AD, Butterbaugh RE, et al. The induction of a cell-mediated immune response to bovine viral diarrhea virus with an adjuvanted inactivated vaccine. Vet Therap 2009;10(4):E1–8.
43. Grooms DL, Coe P. Neutralizing antibody responses in preconditioned calves following vaccination for respiratory viruses. Vet Therap 2002;3(2):119–27.
44. Kerkhofs P, Renjifo X, Toussaint JF, et al. Enhancement of the immune response and virological protection of calves against bovine herpesvirus type 1 with an inactivated gE-deleted vaccine. Vet Rec 2003;152(22):681–6.
45. Walz PH, Givens MD, Rodning SP, et al. Evaluation of reproductive protection against bovine viral diarrhea virus and bovine herpesvirus-1 afforded by annual

revaccination with modified-live viral or combination modified-live/killed viral vaccines after primary vaccination with modified-live viral vaccine. Vaccine 2017;35: 1046–54.

46. Walz PH, Montgomery T, Passler T, et al. Comparison of reproductive performance of primiparous dairy cattle following revaccination with either modified-live or killed multivalent viral vaccines in early lactation. J Dairy Sci 2015;98: 8753–63.

Nutritional Programs for Commercial Replacement Dairy Heifer Operations

A.F. Kertz, Ph.D., DiplACAN

KEYWORDS

- Calves • Milk replacer • Starter • Forage • Water • Rumen development

KEY POINTS

- The goal should be to double calf birth weight at the end of 2 months of life.
- The inverse relationship between milk/milk replacer and starter intakes must be managed to facilitate rumen development and the weaning transition to avoid postweaning slumps.
- Calf starter intake should approximately double each week. Well-texturized starters facilitate rumination, salivation, and functional rumen development without the need for feeding forage and its gut-fill effects.
- Water is the most essential nutrient needed in the greatest quantity by calves. Water is consumed at about 4 times dry matter intake; or if limited, it limits intake and daily gain.
- Warm water should be fed during cold weather so it does not perturb rumen contents temperature and increase calf energy requirements.
- Water and starter should be fed sooner and forage later than the 2014 NAHMS data indicate US dairy producers are doing.

INTRODUCTION

Calves are not born with a functional rumen, so they are initially dependent on a liquid diet. Consumption of the dry starter diet component is the key to functional rumen development, and to allowing calves to be weaned from the liquid diet component. Thus, there is a key interaction between the level of milk/milk replacer (MR) fed and starter consumption. In fact, this is an inverse relationship that must be understood and managed. In an analysis of 9 published studies with 21 treatments,[1] this inverse relationship was quantitated as for each 100 g (0.2 lb) dry matter more milk/MR intake, that decreased starter intake by 60 g (0.13 lb).

There are various calf feeding programs, not simply one, which can be used to double calf birth weight at the end of 2 months of age—the Gold Standard as specified by the Dairy Calf and Heifer Association https://calfandheifer.org/

ANDHIL LLC, 9442 Red vBud Tree Lane, St. Louis, MO 63122, USA
E-mail address: andhil@swbell.net

Vet Clin Food Anim 38 (2022) 39–49
https://doi.org/10.1016/j.cvfa.2021.11.003

TRADITIONAL EARLY WEANING PROGRAM

Origin of an early weaning program was in the 1920s with various Cornell studies.[2] The objective of this program was to curtail costs of milk feeding by weaning early and facilitating rumen development. Whole milk (WM) on the farm was often skimmed off and the fat was used to make butter. The skim milk was then a by-product and often fed to calves or pigs as a MR. Thus, earlier MR made from dried ingredients had what is now considered lower fat content. A 1960 Cornell study[3] used liquid WM, a 2%-nonspecified fat MR, or 25% of either coconut or lard in MRs (dry matter basis). Average daily gains (ADG) were about 0.45 kg (1 lb) and were similar among treatments. That was acknowledged as a satisfactory gain for herd replacements at that time. It was also noted that calves on the 2%-fat MR also ate more calf starter (CS) and thus achieved the same daily gain as the other calves fed higher fat MR or WM.

The 1950s, 1960s, and 1970s were a golden age of studies[4] on rumen development in dairy calves. Studies reviewed[5] in 1979 and a report[6] in 2007 provide good examples of an early weaning program. After the 1970s, MR protein levels progressed down from 22% to 20% and fat levels progressed up from 10 or 12% to 20%. This was related more to marketing and controlling feeding costs with the nutritional benefit being that higher fat levels increased energy intake of calves from MR. But as fat levels increased, MR costs increased, so protein level was also decreased to help offset much of that increased protein cost. Thus, the industry "standard" 20% protein/20% fat MR evolved. But it is erroneous to term that a "standard" as it really became customary or traditional based on how MRs had evolved.

A Minnesota study[7] illustrated that an unintended consequence resulted when fat content was increased in MR (**Table 1**). Higher MR fat at 21% versus 15% resulted in less starter intake and weight gain before weaning, with some carry-over for the 2 weeks after weaning. That is why the 2 weeks after weaning is always critical to measure for carry-over effects from before full weaning. Greater CS intake on the 15.6%-fat MR treatment more than compensated for the reduced metabolizable energy (ME) MR intake on this treatment. The overall effect was 7% more ME intake on the low-fat MR treatment. This similar level (7%) of higher ME intake continued from the CS alone even after calves had been weaned for 14 days. Thus, the greater ME intake from the 21.6% fat MR was more than compensated with reduced CS ME intake resulting in less total energy intake compared with a lower-fat MR treatment. This effect is often unrecognized when high-fat MRs are recommended or fed.

ACCELERATED OR INTENSIVE FEEDING PROGRAM

A paradigm shift occurred in the decade beginning in 2000. Studies at Cornell, Illinois, and Michigan State Universities found that increasing the feeding rate *and* the % protein (CP) in a MR increased daily gain considerably.

Table 1 Calf performance when 15 or 21% fat milk replacers were fed		
% Fat in Milk Replacer	**15**	**21**
Before weaning at 6 wk		
Starter intake, kg (lb)	16.3 (35.9)	12.7 (28.0)
Weight gain, kg (lb)	14.5 (31.9)	11.8 (26.0)
After weaning, 7–8 wk		
Starter intake, kg (lb)	25.9 (57.0)	23.6 (52.0)
Weight gain, kg (lb)	14.4 (31.7)	13.6 (30.0)

But the issue is not just increased weight gain, but what is the composition of that weight gain? Male calves were fed[8] MR differing in fat %, but to gain the same body weight (BW) (**Fig. 1**). Significant differences in body composition resulted. Data were compared on a dry carcass basis because there is an inverse relationship between water and fat in body composition. With 15% fat MR, calves had proportionately more protein and less fat and mineral content compared with 22% and 31% fat MR. No CS was fed to avoid confounding interpreting the results. While this seems counterintuitive, the lowest fat level (15%) MR had the most desirable and appropriate body composition compared with 22% and 31% fat. All three MRs had 28% protein when the ADG was the same among treatments.

In the 2007 National Animal Health Monitoring System (NAHMS) survey, average milk/MR feeding level was 4 quarts (3.78 L) per day with an average weaning age of 8 weeks. In the most recent 2014 NAHMS survey,[9] milk/MR feeding level increased to 6 quarts daily and weaning age increased by 1 week to 9 weeks. That is a 50% increase in milk/MR feeding level. The challenge is to be sure starter intake is adequate and for a long enough time (2–3 weeks) before weaning so that calves do not have a slump in postweaning gain (18%) as noted in Holsteins (**Table 2**) from a 2018 NAHMS study.[10,11]

Various studies[8,12–14] were conducted at Cornell University and at the University of Illinois illustrated the beneficial responses in increased BW gain when MR with higher CP was fed at a higher level than a conventional or traditional MR. The key was to feed

Milk Replacer Fat % Effect on Body Composition

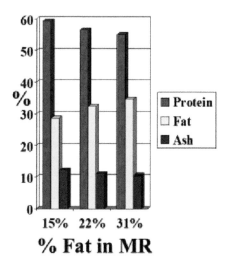

- **Same initial weight**
- **Same ADG ~1.32 lb**
- **Live body weight—fat increased from 8.5 to 11.0%**
- **Result was fatter calves with > 15% fat in MR and also with less protein and mineral content**

Fig. 1. Body composition among milk replacers containing 28% protein but containing 15, 22, or 31% fat when fed for 0.6 kg (1,32 lb) daily gain. (Adapted from Tikofsky, J. N., M. E. Van Amburgh, and D. A. Ross. 2001. Effect of varying carbohydrate and fat. content of milk replacer on body composition of Holstein bull calves. J. Anim. Sci. 79:2260–2267.)

more CP and more MR which did not result in fatter calves as would occur if a 20% CP/20% fat MR was simply fed at similar higher levels. Later, several other studies[15,16] were conducted at Michigan State University. Purchased female Holstein calves[15] were fed for slaughter at either 8 or 14 weeks of age. They were weaned at 7 weeks on trial after having been fed a 20/20 MR at 1.1% of BW reconstituted at 11.8% solids and split into 2 equal feedings, or fed a 28/15 MR at 2% of BW reconstituted at 14.1% solids. Calves remaining after 8 weeks were split further into CS fed at either restricted to achieve 0.4 kg (0.88 lb)/day of ADG or ad libitum with the addition of 30% rolled corn beginning at 9 weeks of age. At 8 weeks, calves gained 0.67 (1.47) versus 0.38 (0.83) kg (lb)/day on 28/15 MR versus 20/20 MR with 2.3 (1 inch) centimeters (cm) more wither height (WH). There were no differences in proportions of water, CP, fat, and ash in carcass between the 2 treatments although carcass weight on the 28/15 MR was 29% greater than on the 20/20 MR. After 8 weeks, the remaining calves were split into either limited or free choice CS treatments within each of the previous 2 to 8-week treatments. At 14 weeks, there were no differences in protein or ash proportions in carcasses, but both ad libitum CS dietary treatments had greater fat content than limited CS diets. Calves fed ad libitum CS exceeded the 1 kg (2.2 lb) ADG, an upper limit target used for identifying undue fattening in calves. The other trial[16] was initiated with similar treatments and MR was fed during the first 6 weeks until weaning at that age, but without restricted CS feeding. Similarly, increased ADG and WH resulted at weaning for 28/15 versus 20/20 MR feeding programs.

How an accelerated MR feeding program performed compared with a traditional MR feeding level and resultant CS intake, ADG, and weaning transition was addressed in another study.[17] In this study, Holstein female and male calves were fed either a conventional 20/20 MR with 12.5% solids at 10% of birth weight daily in 2 feedings from week 1 to 5 and at 5% once daily during week 6; or 28/15 MR with 15% solids at 1.5% of BW as DM during week 1%, 2% of BW as DM during week 2 to 5 divided into 2 daily feedings, and at 5% of BW during week 6 in one daily feeding. All calves were weaned at end of 6 weeks. Feeding less 20/20 MR resulted in greater CS intake ($P < .02$), but less ADG and height increase ($P < .02$) than 28/15 treatments during pre-weaning. Total MR intakes were 19.3 (42.5) for 20/20 and 34.7 (76.4) kg (lb) for 28/15 and 20/20, respectively, with CS intakes before weaning of 14.0 (30.8) and 7.3 (16.1) kg (lb). With greater dry matter intake (DMI) from MR, DMI of CS was reduced on 28/15 MR (**Fig. 2**). But total nutrient intake was greater on 28/15 resulting in greater ADG except for week 7 which was just after full weaning. At the end of 8 weeks, birth BW was approximately doubled on the 28/15 MR treatment, but was about 10 (22.2 lb) kg less on the 20/20 MR treatment. Because of low CS intakes during the first several weeks, some may recommend not feeding the starter at all during the initial weeks. But notice that on both treatments, starter intake approximately doubled from the previous week. If the starter is not fed in the first several weeks, that will shift the intake curve further to the right and result in less total starter intake before full weaning, less starter intake after full weaning, and most likely a slump in ADG as noted in data in **Table 2**.

EFFICIENCIES OF BODY WEIGHT AND HEIGHT GAIN

The requirement for maintenance must be first met before any additional dietary energy can be used for growth, reproduction, or lactation.[18] For a 50 (110 lb) kg calf, the efficiency of ME utilization increases (**Fig. 3**) with increasing daily gain from 21% at 200 (0.44 lb) g/d to 58% at 800 (1.76 lb) g/d. But as a calf grows through the heifer period, its feed efficiency (DM intake/kg ADG) from 1.74 during the first 2 months to

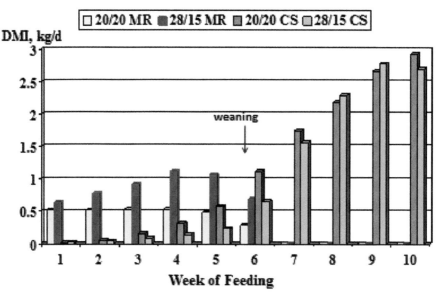

Fig. 2. Milk replacer (MR) and calf starter (CS) dry matter intake (DMI) of calves fed either a 20% CP/20% fat or 28% CP/15% fat MR.[17]

12.6 at about 22 months of age based on data from a large calf/heifer ranch in Spain that I have worked with (A. Bach, personal communication, 2011).

In a Michigan State University study,[15] purchased Holstein heifer calves were fed either 20/20 or 28/15 MR with weaning at 49 days on trial. At the end of 8 weeks on trial, BW, WH, DMI, gain/feed, and cost per kg ADG were all statistically improved by the intensive feeding program (**Table 3**). Body composition analyses found no significant differences in proportions of protein, fat, and ash between the 2 MR treatments. Thus, the additional growth on the intensive MR treatment was not fattening, but true growth.

A similar study[16] with the same treatments was done at Michigan State, but with research herd female calves. After 152 days in their first lactation, net returns per

Table 2		
Extracted from NAHMS 2018 reported data		
Item	Holsteins n = 2273	Jerseys n = 114
Birth weight, kg (lb)	43.0 (94.7)	35.1 (77.3)
Weaning weight, kg (lb)	91.4 (201.3)	70.1 (154.4)
Daily gain, kg (lb)	**0.73 (1.61)**	0.51 (1.12)
90-d weight, kg (lb)	104.0 (229.0)	86.2 (189.8)
Daily gain postweaned, kg (lb)	**0.60 (1.32)**	0.76 (1.69)
Birth hip height, cm (inch)	82.8 (32.6)	75.7 (29.8)
Weaning hip height, cm (inch)	95.3 (37.5)	85.6 (33.7)
Cm (inch)/day	0.18 (0.071)	0.145 (0.057)
90-d hip height, cm (inch)	98.0 (38.6)	89.9 (35.4)
Inch/mo	5.11 (2.01)	4.75 (1.87)

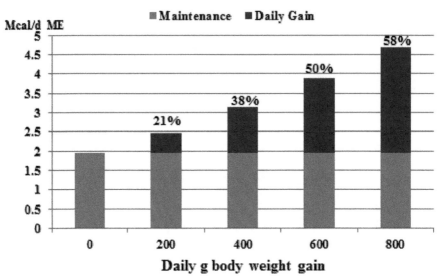

Fig. 3. Efficiency (%) of metabolizable energy (ME) utilization with increasing rates of daily gain by 50 kg calf.

treatment were $83 for conventional and $170 for intensive fed calves. The $53 more feed cost per calf for the intensive treatment returned an additional $87 more through just the first 152 days in the calf's first lactation. In a detailed economic comparison of conventional versus intensive calf programs, the net return[19] through first lactation (including that milk response determined by a Cornell study[20]) was $205 more for Intensive versus conventional MR programs.

CALF STARTERS

Extensive rumen development studies were conducted in the 1950s to 1970s at Iowa State, Cornell, and the United Kingdom National Institute for Research in Dairying. Several studies, such as in this one,[21] determined that "these data confirm the view that end-products of rumen fermentation rather than the coarse nature of the feed

Table 3
Performance of calves fed either conventional or intensive milk replacer programs at the end of 8 wk on trial.[15]

	Conventional	Intensive
Initial body weight, kg (lb)	44.1 (97.1)	44.0 (96.9)
8-wk weight, kg (lb)	60.0^a (92.1)	72.1^b (58.8)
Wither height, cm (inch)	77.4^a (30.5)	78.1^b (30.7)
8-wk height, cm (inch)	83.5^a (32.9)	85.9^b (33.8)
DM starter intake, kg (lb)/day	0.41^a (0.90)	0.34^b (0.75)
Total DMI, kg (lb)/day	0.85^a (1.87)	1.21^b (2.66)
Gain/feed	0.44^a	0.55^b
$/kg gain (lb)	2.88^a (1.31)	2.73^b (1.24)

$^{a,b}P < .05$ difference between both treatments.

are the stimuli for the development of rumen papillae." In another study,[22] infused acetate, propionate, butyrate, glucose, and sodium chloride at feeding time into 2 rumen-fistulated calves/treatment of 11 weeks until sacrificed at ~100 days age helped determine that volatile fatty acids (VFA) stimulated rumen papillae development in the order of butyric > propionic > acetic. After calves had been weaned early,[23] and fed a diet with either 90% concentrate or 90% hay, daily gains were 0.5 kg (1.1 lb) or 0.3 kg (0.66 lb), respectively, with the latter calves described as being "thin, pot-bellied, and unthrifty". This reduced ADG and increased gut fill were demonstrated[24] when calves were fed on various treatments after weaning diets with concentrate fixed at 0.45 (1.0), 0.91 (2.0), 1.36 (3.0), 1.82 (4.0), or 2.25 (5.0) kg (lb) daily with corresponding free choice hay intakes being 61%, 31%, 25%, 16%, and 4% of total DMI. Daily gain increased to about 0.60 (1.3) kg (lb) somewhat linearly along with corresponding rumen papillae development as concentrate intake increased. This ADG occurred at 16% and 4% hay in total DMI. But results were confounded as gut contents increased with increasing hay intakes. Thus, the best ADG, rumen papillae development, and least gut fill occurred with the highest concentrate/lowest hay intakes. Unfortunately, more recent CS studies in which hay is fed do not measure gut fill and implicitly assume there is no difference or that it is immaterial. That is not a safe assumption.

In the early 1970s, a study[6] was conducted in which CSs were formulated with 2 levels of fiber and 2 physical forms of meal versus mash (texturized). While there were some differences due to fiber level, the greatest differences were due to the physical form of the starter. But what is a properly texturized starter? That study[6] contains particle size data for reference as did another study[25] which found negative effects for calves when including hay in a well-texturized starter. In a further study,[26] negative effects were found for fines/small particles on starter intake and ADG. There are also extensive data on CS particle size distributions along with ingredient and nutrient composition in this report of 5 calf trials. In general, more than 45% of the formulation needs to come from corn, oats, or barley which can be whole (except for barley), rolled, or cracked.

Fermentation is required in the calf rumen to initiate rumen papillae development. These papillae in turn absorb the VFA as the calf's primary energy source. The key is to have a fermentation that enhances butyrate production and secondarily propionate, because both these VFAs are most stimulatory for rumen papillae development. Ruminal acidosis limits intake and reduces digestibility.[6] Well-texturized starters work because that leads to calves ruminating more. This results in more saliva production that buffers the rumen from becoming too acidotic. Pelleted starters do not have particle size to aid this process. Hay or roughage would need to be fed to avoid that acidosis,[27] but then this does not help produce the optimal pattern of butyrate and propionate in rumen fermentation. And that type of fermentation does not facilitate rumen papillae development. The best illustration of this is to view slides on this Penn State website link. http://extension.psu.edu/animals/dairy/health/nutrition/calves/calf-rumen-images Calves on a pelleted starter can be heard or seen at times trying to compensate for this problem by chewing loudly on wood. This facilitates salivation which helps buffer their too acidotic rumen.

A study[28] which illustrates several issues discussed fed calves a starter described as "texturized" alone or with hay. The starter had "14% flatted barley, 13% flatted oats, and 10% steamed corn" which summed to 37% processed grains. Except for barley, it is not usually necessary to process grains for a texturized starter. But the low rumen pH of 5.06 (**Table 4**) clearly shows that starter alone treatment was not adequately texturized. As BWs were not different between the 2 treatments, true BW was distorted by 4.7 (10.4) kg (lb) more gut fill (0.32 kg or 0.7 lb of that could

Table 4
Effect of hay intake along with starter on gut fill.[28]

	Starter	Starter/ Hay	P <
Rumen-reticulum + digesta, kg (lb)	8.0 (17.6)	12.7 (28.0)	0.02
Rumen-reticulum – digesta, kg (lb)	1.6 (3.5)	1.9 (4.2)	0.03
Rumen pH	5.06	5.49	0.002

have been from the increased tissue weight too) on the starter/hay treatment. This gut fill may not likely be visually evident. Thus, calf trials in which hay is or is not fed, such as in this trial, should have gut fill measurements to not have confounded growth data.

FEEDING WATER

Water is the nutrient needed in the greatest quantity by calves. It is consumed at about 4 times DMI,[29] as is also true for heifers and cows. Two very practical dimensions of feeding water to calves are, first, to be sure there is adequate separation between water and starter containers so calves do not drop water into starter and vice versa and reduce intake of both (**Table 5**). Water needs to be provided to encourage calves to eat starter earlier. In another study,[30] waiting until 17 days after birth to begin feeding water to calves did not have major effects on starter intake and performance; most likely due to high milk feeding levels (6–9 L daily) and subsequent lower starter intake. But postweaning (50–70 days), calves had greater hip height, body length, ADF and NDF digestibilities, and feed efficiency when feeding water began right after birth. And at 5 months of age, these calves had 13.2 kg (29 lb) more BW.

The other dimension is that calves like warm water, especially in colder weather. In one study,[31] it required around an hour for the rumen temperature of calves to return to near normal following a 6.6 °C (20°F) drop after calves drank 8 °C (46.4°) water. Drinking water of 17.2 (63), 27.2 (81), and 37.2° (99°F) temperatures produced progressively lesser rumen temperature drops, but it still required about an hour for rumen temperatures to return to near normal. Another benefit of warm water feeding is that during winter, calves would not need to use additional energy to warm colder water to rumen temperature; and a 3rd water feeding can help increase starter intake and its subsequent heat of rumen fermentation to keep warmer.

FIELD PRACTICES

There was little difference between when US dairy producers began first feeding water in the 2014[9] versus 2007 NAHMS databases. In 2014, the average age was 17 days (**Fig. 4**). That is part of the unfortunate picture in which dairy producers wait too long to begin feeding water and starter but cannot wait to begin feeding hay too soon—and the picture is worst for smaller dairy farms. The average age at weaning

Table 5
Calf performance for the month postweaned following an early weaning program when water and starter were adjacent or separated

2nd Month of age	Separated	Adjacent
Weight gain, kg (lb)/d	0.84 (1.85)	0.72 (1.59)
Starter intake, kg (lb)/d	2.28 (5.02)	2.02 (4.85)
Water intake, kg (kg)/d	8.20 (18.1)	6.20 (13.7)

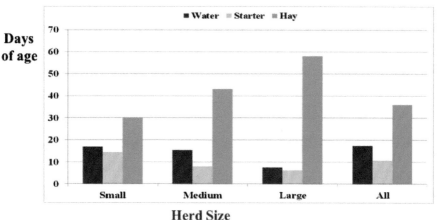

Fig. 4. Calf age when dairy producers began first feeding water, starter, and hay according to 2014 NAHMS data.[9]

increased from 8 weeks in 2007 to 9 weeks in 2014. This was undoubtedly due to the daily feeding rate of milk/MR increasing from 4 quarts to 6 quarts—a 50% increase. The direct relationship between water and starter intake indicates water and starter should be fed beginning within days after birth, and forage should not be fed at all until after weaning when fed a well-texturized starter or limited to 5% when fed with a meal or pelleted starter.

CLINICS CARE POINTS

- Evaluate and determine milk/milk replacer feeding program.
- Evaluate type of starter being fed and its typical intakes.
- Determine weaning program followed especially during transition 2 weeks before and 2 weeks after full weaning to avoid postweaning slump.
- Evaluate water feeding program, that starter and water containers are physically separate to avoid cross-contamination, and that warm water is fed during cold weather.
- Confirm that water and starter feeding begins after colostrum/transition milk feeding, and that forage is not fed until after weaning unless a meal or all pelleted starter is being fed.

DISCLOSURE

The author has nothing to disclose.

REFERENCES

1. Gelsinger SL, Heinrichs AJ, Jones CM. A meta-analysis of the effects of pre-weaned calf nutrition and growth on first-lactation performance. J Dairy Sci 2016;99:6206–14.

2. Kertz AF, Hill TM, Quigley JD III, et al. Calf nutrition and management: a 100-year historical review. J Dairy Sci 2017;100:10151–72.

3. Kertz AF, Loften JR. A historical perspective and brief review: holstein dairy calf milk replacer feeding programs in the. U.S Prof Anim Scientist 2013;29:321–32.

4. Kertz AF. Dairy calf and heifer feeding and management—some key concepts and practices. outskirts press,157. 2019. Available at: https://outskirtspress.com/dairycalfandheiferfeedingandmanagement and also. available from Amazon, and Barnes & Noble.

5. Kertz AF, Prewitt LR, Everett JP Jr. An early weaning calf program: summarization and review. J Dairy Sci 1979;62:1835–43.

6. Porter JC, Warner RG, Kertz AF. Effect of fiber level and physical form of starter on growth and development of dairy calves fed no forage. Prof Anim Scientist 2007;23:395–400.

7. Kuehn CS, Otterby DE, Linn JG, et al. The effect of dietary energy concentration on calf performance. J Dairy Sci 1994;77:2621–9.

8. Tikofsky JN, Van Amburgh ME, Ross DA. Effect of varying carbohydrate and fat content of milk replacer on body composition of Holstein bull calves. J Anim Sci 2001;79:2260–7.

9. National Animal Health Monitoring System. Dairy 2014. Dairy Cattle Management Practices in the United Sates. United States Dept. of Agric., Animal Plant and Health Inspection Service, Veterinary Services, February 2016, Fort Collins, CO. https://www.aphis.usda.gov/animal_health/nahms/dairy/downloads/dairy14/Dairy14_dr_Mastitis.pdf

10. Urie NJ, Lombard JE, Shivley CB, et al. Preweaned heifer management on US dairy operations: Part I. Descriptive characteristics of preweaned heifer raising practices. J Dairy Sci 2018a;101:9168–84.

11. Urie NJ, Lombard JE, Shivley CB, et al. Preweaned heifer management on US dairy operations: Part V. Factors associated with morbidity and mortality in pre-weaned dairy heifer calves. J Dairy Sci 2018b;101:9229–44.

12. Diaz MC, Van Amburgh ME, Smith JM, et al. Composition of growth of Holstein calves fed milk replacer from birth to 105-kilogram body weight. J Dairy Sci 2001;84:830–42.

13. Blome RM, Drackley JK, McKeith FK, et al. Growth, nutrient utilization, and body composition of dairy calves fed milk replacers containing different amounts of protein. J Anim Sci 2003;81:1641–55.

14. Bartlett KS, McKeith FK, VandeHaar MJ, et al. Growth and body composition of dairy calves fed milk replacers containing different amounts of protein at two feeding rates. J Anim Sci 2006;84:1454–67.

15. Brown EG, VandeHaar MJ, Daniels KM, et al. Effect of increasing energy and protein intake on body growth and carcass composition of heifer calves. J Dairy Sci 2005;88:585–94.

16. Davis Rincker LE, VandeHaar MJ, Wolf CA, et al. Effect of intensified feeding of heifer calves on growth, pubertal age, calving age, milk yield, and economics. J Dairy Sci 2011;94:3554–67, 95:783-793.

17. Stamey JA, Janovick NA, Kertz AF, et al. Influence of starter protein content on growth of dairy calves in an enhanced early nutrition program. J.Dairy Sci 2012;95:3327–36.

18. NRC. 2001. Nutrient requirements of dairy Cattle. 7th rev. edition. Washington, DC: National Academy Press; 2001.

19. Overton MW, Corbett RB, Boomer WG. An economic comparison of conventional vs, intensive heifer rearing. Proc West. Dairy Management Conf. 2013;123–31.

20. Soberon F, Raffrenato E, Everett RW, et al. Preweaning milk replacer intake and effects on long term productivity of dairy calves. J Dairy Sci 2012;95:783–93.
21. Flatt WP, Warner RG, Loosli JK. Influence of purified materials on the development of the ruminant stomach. J Dairy Sci 1958;41:1593–600.
22. Sander EG, Warner RG, Harrison HN, et al. The stimulatory effect of sodium butyrate and sodium propionate on the development of rumen mucosa in the young calf. J Dairy Sci 1959;42:1600–5.
23. Harrison HN, Warner RG, Sander EG, et al. Changes in the tissue and volume of the stomachs of calves following the removal of dry feed or consumption of inert bulk. J Dairy Sci 1960;43:1301–12.
24. Stobo IJF, Roy JHB, Gaston HJ. Rumen development in the calf. I. The effect of diets containing different proportions of concentrates to hay on rumen development. Br J Nut 1966;20:171–92.
25. Hill TM, Bateman HG II, Aldrich JM, et al. Effects of the amount of chopped hay or cottonseed hull in a textured calf starter on young calf performance. J Dairy Sci 2008;91:2684–93.
26. Bateman HG II, Hill TM, et al. Effects of corn processing, particle size, and diet form on performance of calves in bedded pens. J Dairy Sci 2009;92:782–9.
27. Terre M, Pedrals E, Dalmau A, et al. What do preweaned and weaned calves need in the diet: A high fiber content or a forage source? J Dairy Sci 2013;96: 5217–26.
28. Khan MA, Weary DM, von Keyserlingk MAG. Hay intake improves performance and rumen development of calves fed higher quantities of milk. J Dairy Sci 2011;94:3547–53.
29. Kertz AF, Reutzel LF, Mahoney JH. Ad libitum water intake by neonatal calves and its relationship to calf starter Intake, weight gain, feces score, and season. J Dairy Sci 1984;67:2964–9.
30. Wickramasinghe J, Kramer AJ, Appuhamy JADRN. Drinking water intake of newborn dairy calves and its effects on feed intake, growth performance, health status, and nutrient digestibility. J Dairy Sci 2019;102:377–87.
31. Dracy AE, Kurtenbach AJ. Temperature change within the rumen, crop area, and rectal area when liquid of various temperature was fed to calves. J Dairy Sci 1968;51:1787–90.

Modeling Preweaning Dairy Calf Performance

Rich Larson, DVM, PhD*

KEYWORDS

• Modeling • Preweaning • Growth • calf nutrition

KEY POINTS

- Concerted research efforts to ascertain the underlying mechanisms associated with and factors affecting body composition and weight gain during the preweaning phase have led to the development of a modeling construct for young calf growth.
- Factors including plane of nutrition (ie, protein and fat), breed of calf, and environmental conditions can be modeled to estimate and compare body weight gain between differing feeding programs.
- The relationship between liquid and dry feed intakes needs to be more clearly defined over a wider range of liquid feed intakes so the impact on growth during weaning and post-weaning can be more accurately assessed.

INTRODUCTION

Nutrition and growth of the dairy calf through weaning has evolved beyond the "one size fits all" approach. Historically dairy calves have been fed a "conventional" feeding program, whereby whole milk/milk replacer is limited fed during the liquid feeding phase to typically 0.08 to 0.10 of body weight as liquid ($\sim$1.0 lb (0.454 KG) solids/head/d) in an effort to encourage consumption of dry starter feeds and earlier weaning. This approach to feeding dairy calves has differed from nursery feeding practices in other sectors of the animal livestock world, whereby ad libitum intakes of nutrients are the norm and lead to more biologically allowable growth during the early life of the animal.

There have been many technologies used and much research conducted in the last 10 to 20 years that has led to feeding strategies providing an increased plane of nutrition to nursery calves. Some of these innovations include:

1. Proliferation of on-farm milk pasteurizers, leading to increased supply and utilization of nonsalable milk to feed to calves.
2. Increased use of automatic calf feeders, allowing for more frequent and larger volumes of nutrients to be delivered to the young calf.

Cud Bud Enterprises, LLC. 1104 Palmer Dr. Laramie, WY 82070, USA
* Corresponding author.
E-mail address: cklhawk@frontiernet.net

Vet Clin Food Anim 38 (2022) 51–62
https://doi.org/10.1016/j.cvfa.2021.11.004
0749-0720/22/© 2021 Elsevier Inc. All rights reserved.
vetfood.theclinics.com

3. Research into how feeding the young dairy heifer calf affects body composition and mammary development during the early growth period along with impacts on later-life health, productivity, and longevity.
4. Paired- and group-housing of calves leading to labor efficiencies, less stressful weaning, and increased ability of calves to adapt to novel situations.

The industry as a whole has migrated from these historical conventional feeding rates to adopting feeding practices with increased daily feeding rates ($\geq$ 1.25 lb (0.567 KG) solids/head/d) and increased milk replacer crude protein contents ($\geq$ 22%). The new normal has become "moderate" and "intensive" or "accelerated" feeding programs designed to increase the supply of energy and protein to meet the maintenance needs associated with the basic metabolic functions of life, to regulate body temperature outside the calf's thermoneutral zone (cold and heat stress), to provide increased energy to the immune system in response to disease challenges as well as the stressors associated with transportation and new surroundings, and to support an acceptable rate of growth during the nursery phase. In addition, feeding programs will include step-up procedures during the first 2 weeks of the liquid feeding phase to minimize digestive upsets as well as step-down procedures before weaning to minimize decreases in postweaning performance as the calf transitions to becoming a fully functional ruminant. All of these factors contribute to creating site-specific feeding programs based on the goals and objectives of the calf raising operation (eg, dairy heifer replacements vs dairy beef).

Some historical growth rates associated with conventional, modified, and intensive nutritional programs are shown in **Table 1**.[1] In a more recent review of research conducted at the Nurture Research Center Data (Provimi US), a comprehensive data analysis on 491 calves across 10 published studies was used to examine the effects of moderate or high milk replacer feeding rates on growth performance through 56 days of the nursery feeding period (**Table 2**).[2] In a summary of more than 1200 dairy heifer calves fed an intensive feeding program (28% CP–15% fat or 28% CP–20% fat milk replacers fed at 2%–2.5% of birth weight) at the Cornell University Teaching and Research dairy herd, calves had a mean preweaning average daily gain of 1.81 lb/d (0.82 kg/d).[3] As a point of reference, a study conducted by von Keyserlingk and colleagues showed Holstein heifer calves fed whole milk on an ad lib basis averaged approximately 2.4 lb/d (1.1 kg/d).[4]

Table 1
Expected average growth rates for calves of various ages under different nutritional programs

	Expected Growth Rate	
Feeding Program & Stage	**lb/d**	**kg/d**
Conventional, ad libitum starter, d 0–42[a] (Typically, 1.00 lb solids/hd/d of a 20% CP, 20% Fat MR)	1.10–1.32	0.5–0.6
Moderate, ad libitum starter, d 0–42[c] (1.25–2.0 lb solids/hd/d of a 22%–25% CP, 18%–20% Fat MR)	1.21–1.43	0.55–0.65
Accelerated, ad libitum starter, d 0–42[b] (Typically, 2.25 lb solids/hd/d of a 28% CP, 15%–20% Fat MR)	1.32–1.76	0.6–0.8
Weaned calves, ad libitum starter, < 1.1 lb/d forage, d 56–84	1.87–2.09	0.85–0.95

[a] Gains during d 0–21 would be 0.44–0.66 lb/d (0.2–0.3 kg/d)
[b] Gains during d 0–21 would be 1.10–1.32 lb/d (0.5–0.6 kg/d)
[c] Gains during d 0–21 would be 0.88–1.10 lb/d (0.4–0.5 kg/d)
    Data from Drackley, JK. Calf Nutrition from Birth to Breeding. Vet Clin Food Anim 2008;24:55-86.

Developing modeling programs for complex biologic functions such as milk production or growth are done under controlled conditions in experimental settings to limit as many external variables as possible. Caution is advised when applying modeling programs in commercial settings as multiple external factors not included in the development of the modeling equations may have an impact on the results obtained. For example, lack of colostrum feeding practices and subsequent exposure to infectious disease can have profound impacts on calf performance as energy is diverted from body weight gain to fueling the immune system. In addition, comparing modeling results between calf raising operations with differing management practices not directly related to nutrition may lead to different findings. But within a calf raising operation, making comparisons using modeling concepts can provide value when evaluating different feeding programs that provide differing planes of nutrition (ie, moderate vs accelerated feeding) or under different environmental conditions (ie, cold stress).

This article will provide some background on the development and existence of calf growth modeling principles and consider some of the variables that have been shown to have an impact on the energy and protein requirements of the young calf.

BACKGROUND
NRC 2001 calf submodel

The 2001 NRC (National Research Council Nutrient Requirements of Dairy Cattle)[5] devoted an entire chapter to the nutrient requirements of the young calf. In addition to reviewing and updating the nutrient requirements of the young calf with the latest research available at the time, a section of the software associated with the publication was used to model the energy and protein requirements during the liquid feeding phase.

The Young Calf Sub-Model within the NRC 2001 software introduced the concept of energy allowable growth (EAG) and protein allowable growth (PAG). A summary of the energy allowable gain calculations is as follows:

(1) Basal maintenance requirement of the calf without stress is calculated based on body weight.

Table 2
Performance of calves fed moderate or high rates of milk replacer (MR) in the nursery period (day 0–56).

Parameter	Moderate MR[a]	High MR[b]
Initial Body Weight, lb	93.0	95.2
ADG, lb/d	1.21	1.39
Gain/DMI, lb/lb	.466	.488
MR Intake, lb/d (DM basis)	1.03	1.77
Starter Intake, lb/d (DM basis)	1.53	1.04

[a] Moderate MR = 1.41 to 1.46 lb DM/d for the first 35 to 39 d, followed by half the allotment per day for 3 to 7 d.
[b] High MR = 2.03 to 2.36 lb DM/d for the first 35 to 44 d, followed by half the allotment per day for 5 to 7 d.
Data from Hu et al. Effects of milk replacer feeding rates on growth performance of Holstein dairy calves to 4 months of age, evaluated via a meta-analytical approach. J Dairy Sci 2020; 013:2217-2232.

(2) If the calf is subjected to cold stress, an additional multiplier factor is applied to the basal maintenance requirement based on the ambient temperature to which the calf is exposed.

(3) The total amount energy available in the diet is calculated.

    a. The metabolizable energy (ME), net energy maintenance (NEm), and net energy gain (NEg) values for the individual feeds in the diet are calculated. Various efficiency factors are used to proceed through the energy cascade calculations for ME, NEm, and NEg based on the type of feed used in the diet (whole milk/milk replacer vs dry feed (eg, calf starter, calf grower).

    b. A composite ME, NEm, and NEg for the diet is calculated based on the individual dry matter (DM) contributions of the individual feeds to the overall diet.

(4) The NEm requirement of the calf and the NEm concentration of the diet are used to calculate the diet DM amount needed to meet the calf's maintenance requirement.

(5) Any additional diet DM available after meeting the calf NEm requirement along with the NEg concentration of the diet is used to calculate the EAG value.

Protein allowable gain calculations are as follows

(1) An apparently digestible protein (ADP) maintenance requirement is calculated based on endogenous losses through urine and feces.

(2) The total amount of ADP supply in the diet is calculated based on the individual DM contributions of the individual feeds in the diet, their crude protein concentrations, and crude protein to ADP efficiency factors.

(3) The ADP maintenance requirement is subtracted from the ADP supply, and any remaining surplus is used to calculate the PAG value.

The NRC 2001 Calf Sub-Model allows for inputs of calf body weight, temperature, and individual feeds and amounts comprising the diet for a single point in time. The model allows for differences in body weight, rate of gain, and environmental temperatures to be used in determining nutrient requirements. Providing estimates of EAG and PAG were a huge step forward in understanding the energy and protein requirements at various calf weights/ages. For example, cold stress has the impact of increasing the energy maintenance requirement of the calf and decreasing the amount of energy left over to go toward gain if the energy content of the diet is not increased. This is especially evident during the first 3 weeks of age, when calves are at increased susceptibility to cold stress.

Cornell–Illinois equations

In the early 2000s after the publication of the 2001 NRC Nutrient Requirements of Dairy Cattle, much research was devoted to the underlying physiology of young calf growth, specifically how feeding differing amounts of dietary energy and protein to the young calf affected overall body composition. Research by Diaz,[6] Tikofsky,[7] Blome et. al,[8] and Bartlett and colleagues[9] provided a large data set that led to a better understanding of the ME and crude protein requirements of dairy calves. Subsequently, these data allowed the development of the Cornell–Illinois equations which provided an update to the NRC 2001 Calf Sub-Model. **Table 3**[10] shows the effect of these modifications, with the modified equations resulting in slightly lower values for ME and slightly higher values for crude protein when compared with NRC 2001 estimates.

Agricultural Modeling & Training Systems Calf Model

Agricultural Modeling & Training Systems (AMTS) have incorporated growth modeling for the preweaned calf into their commercially available AMTS.Farm.Cattle Pro ration

Table 3
Comparison of nutrient requirements for a 50-kg calf between 2001 NRC and Cornell–Illinois equations (thermoneutral conditions).[1]

Rate of gain, lb/ d (kg/d)	Dry matter intake, % BW	Metabolizable energy, Mcal/d		Crude protein, gm/d		Crude protein, % of diet dry matter	
		NRC 2001	Cornell-Illinois	NRC 2001	Cornell-Illinois	NRC 2001	Cornell-Illinois
0.44 (0.20)	1.05	2.37	2.34	78	94	18.7	18.0
0.88 (0.4)	1.30	3.00	2.89	125	150	21.4	22.4
1.32 (0.6)	1.57	3.70	3.49	173	207	23.7	26.6
1.76 (0.8)	1.84	4.46	4.40	220	253	25.1	27.4
2.20 (1.0)	2.30	5.25	4.80	267	318	26.1	28.6

Adapted from Drackley, JK. Calf Nutrition from Birth to Breeding. Vet Clin Food Anim 2008;24:55-86.

formulation program.[11] The modeling incorporates the underlying concepts of the NRC 2001 Calf Sub-Model, updated information from the Cornell-Illinois Equations (discussed above), and internal AMTS development. The AMTS Calf Model allows for multiple animal (breed, age, weight) and environmental inputs to define the nutrient requirements of the calf along with a dedicated feed library designed for use in non-ruminating, milk-fed calves. More information is available at https:// agmodelsystems.com/.

Milk Specialties Global Toolkit Calf Growth Model

Milk Specialties Global (MSG), a manufacturer of milk replacers for the dairy industry, has developed a web-based calf growth modeling program (https://toolkit. milkspecialties.com/). This commercially available program is viewable across multiple formats (Android and Apple) and multiple devices (laptop, tablet, and phone).

Whereas the NRC 2001 Calf Sub-Model program evaluates calf growth at a single point in time, the MSG Calf Growth Model is unique in that it evaluates calf growth over an entire feeding period. The program uses the basic concepts outlined in the NRC 2001 Calf Sub-Model, calculating an energy allowable gain, protein allowable gain, and an average daily gain (ADG) for each day of the feeding period based on user inputs. User inputs include breed of calf, starting weight, temperature, and feeding period length. The diet inputs can consist of multiple feeds that are components of the liquid diet (eg, milk replacer, whole milk) and of the dry diet (ie, calf starter). For each feed, the user enters an average daily consumption on a weekly basis. For liquid diet feeds, the program uses the same inputted value for each day of the week (ie, 1.25 lb/hd/d of milk replacer) (0.567 KG/hd/d of milk replacer). For dry diet feeds, the program performs a regression analysis of the inputted weekly values to calculate a daily feed consumption across the entire feeding period. Multiple result parameters can be selected and are presented in graphical and tabular formats on the web-based platform. As new information on young calf growth is continuously being generated, refer to the User Guide on the website for the latest information on the underlying principles and calculations associated with the MSG Calf Growth Model.

National Academies of Science, Engineering, and Medicine Dairy 2021

The National Academies of Science, Engineering, and Medicine (NASEM) is expected to release an updated Nutrient Requirements for Dairy Cattle in the latter half of 2021.

This publication will provide updated concepts and equations for the energy and protein requirements of the young calf based on research conducted since the NRC 2001 Nutrient Requirements of Dairy Cattle. In addition to including more refined estimations of calf growth during the preweaning period, this publication will provide prediction equations for starter intake based on calf body weight and energy consumption from the liquid diet as well as an updated software program for modeling young calf growth. This author refers you to the AMTS and MSG Toolkit websites for updates on incorporation of the calf growth modeling concepts from the NASEM publication's official release.

GROWTH MODEL CONSIDERATIONS
Cold stress and heat stress

The thermoneutral temperature range for young-adapted calves is estimated to be 59° to 77° F (15°–25° C) (Van Amburgh[10]). For cold stress, the lower critical temperature (LCT) of 59° F (15° C) is most appropriate for the young calf in the first 3 weeks of age. The LCT decreases with increasing body weight and age and is approximated to be 41° F (5° C) for calves older than 3 weeks of age through weaning. The NRC 2001 Calf Sub-Model used a stair-step approach to estimating the increase in maintenance requirement for the young calf, applying multiplier factors for various temperature ranges below the LCT (**Table 4**). In place of this stair-step approach, the MSG Calf Growth Model and AMTS Calf Model apply an adjustment factor for every degree below the LCT based on a regression analysis. The impact of cold stress on the calf growth is most noticeable in the calf less than 3 weeks of age as calves are born with limited energy stores and minimal consumption of dry feed is not providing much additional energy to the diet. Cold stress does not appear to impact the calf's protein requirement to any large degree.

Heat stress has a negative impact on average daily gain and calf performance. In a 2006 study conducted by Wiedmeier and colleagues[12] that considered the effects of season, preweaning average daily gain of calves started in June was lowest (1.39 lb/d)

Table 4
Multiplier factors applied to the maintenance requirement for young calves exposed to cold stress

Temp° F	Temp° C	Calves < 3 wk of age	Calves > 3 wk of age
> 59	> 15	1.00	1.00
50–59	10–15	1.13	1.00
41–50	5–10	1.27	1.00
32–41	0–5	1.40	1.13
23–32	−5 to 0	1.54	1.27
14–23	−10 to −5	1.68	1.40
5–14	−15 to −10	1.86	1.54
−4 to 5	−20 to −15	1.94	1.68
−13 to −4	−25 to −20	2.08	1.81
−22 to −13	−30 to −25	2.21	1.94
< −22	< −30	2.34	2.07

Data from National Research Council. Nutrient requirements of dairy cattle. 7th edition. Washington, DC: National Academy Press; 2001.

(0.631 kg/d), whereas the average daily gain of calves started in September and March was highest (1.55 and 1.53 lb/d) (0.704 and 0.695 kg/d), respectively). Calves started in December had an intermediate average daily gain (1.46 lb/d) (0.663 KG/d). Place and colleagues[13] also found lower average daily gains in calves born in summer and fall. A review by Chester-Jones et al.[14] of data on over 2800 Holstein calves from 2004 to 2012 also showed that birth season had an effect on average daily gain, with calves born in the summer averaging significantly less (1.37 lb/d) (0.622 kg/d) than calves born in fall and winter (1.46 lb/d) (0.663 kg/d). The energetic costs of heat stress on calf performance have not yet been quantified in an experimental setting to the level that has been done for cold stress. The AMTS Calf Model applies the same regression logic used for calculating cold stress maintenance energy increases to the heat stress side of the thermo-neutral zone for young calves.

Breed differences

A majority of the research done to elucidate the underlying physiology of young calf growth has been conducted on large breed calves (Holsteins). Small breed or Jersey calves have a greater surface area to body weight relationship, which translates to a greater heat loss potential. Research at Virginia Tech (Bascom[15]) on Jersey calves showed the maintenance energy requirements of Jersey calves are higher than for Holstein calves and most likely need to be fed higher fat diets. Both the AMTS Calf Model and MSG Calf Growth Model provide the option to select the breed of calf being fed and make an appropriate adjustment to the maintenance energy requirements in the model.

Calf starter intake

Several studies have demonstrated the inverse relationship between liquid and dry feed intakes during the preweaning phase of the feeding program for a young calf.[2,16,17] A meta-analysis of the effects of preweaned calf nutrition and growth on first-lactation performance by Gelsinger and colleagues[18,] showed a strong inverse relationship between liquid and starter intakes (**Fig. 1**). This is most likely due to the calf's limited capacity for daily DM intake. This correlation was especially strong when the liquid feed DM feeding rate was greater than 1.76 lb/d (0.8 kg/d). Starter DM intake was more variable at lower liquid feed DM intakes.

When modeling a particular feeding program, accurate determinations of liquid and dry feed intakes are essential. In most situations, liquid feeding rates will be more easily known, either because restricted amounts are being offered and consumed or in robotic feeding situations, the amounts consumed are being recorded. Conversely, dry starter feed is generally offered on an ad-libitum basis and ascertaining actual consumption can be difficult to obtain or is not routinely tracked on commercial calf raising operations. Under research settings, however, actual daily dry starter intakes can be accurately determined under differing liquid feeding rates (**Fig. 2**).[2] This can lead to mathematical representations and regression equations being developed for dry starter intakes during the nursery phase that can be used as a basis in calf growth modeling. Data from 2 experiments at the Martin Experiment Station, Martin TN from 1992 to 1993 were used to develop a regression equation to predict calf starter DM intake in calves fed commercial milk replacer and calf starter.[19] Significant variables in the determination of calf starter intake included calf sex, age, body weight, average daily gain, and milk replacer DM intake. However, this regression analysis was limited due to the upper limit of milk replacer fed (1.9 lb/d or 0.86 kg/d). Updated regression analyses are needed to predict calf starter intake over a wider range of liquid feeding rates.

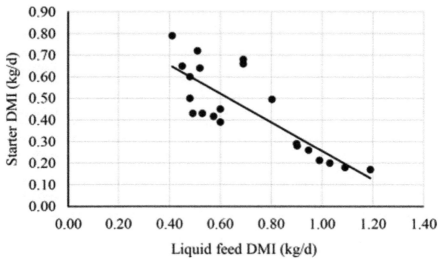

Fig. 1. Relationship ($r = -0.82$; $Y = -0.66X + 0.92$) between daily DMI before weaning as liquid feed (milk of milk replacer) and as starter grain. Each data point represents 1 of 21 treatments from 9 individual studies comparing preweaned calf management with first-lactation performance. (*Data from* Gelsinger et al. A meta-analysis of the effects of preweaned calf nutrition and growth on first lactation performance. J Dairy Sci 2016;99:6206-6214.)

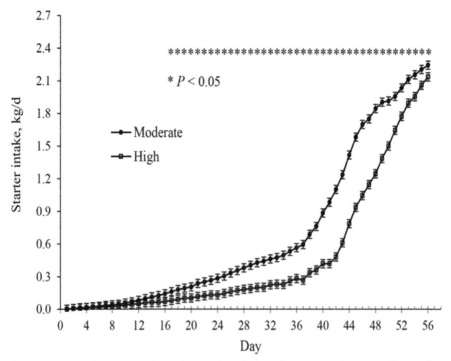

Fig. 2. Starter intake pattern for Holstein calves fed moderate rates (1.41–1.46 lb DM/d) or high rates (2.03–2.36) of milk replacer in the nursery period. Asterisks indicate that starter intake at the same week differed in the calves fed moderate versus high rates of milk replacer ($P < .05$). (*Data from* Hu et al. Effects of milk replacer feeding rates on growth performance of Holstein dairy calves to 4 months of age, evaluated via a meta-analytical approach. J Dairy 2020;013:2217-2232.)

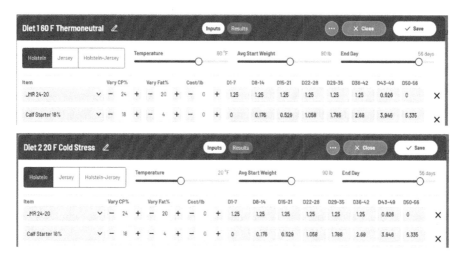

Fig. 3. Data inputs for the comparison of calf growth performance between thermoneutral (60° F) and cold stress conditions (20° F) using the Milk Specialties Global Calf Growth Model (https://toolkit.milkspecialties.com/).

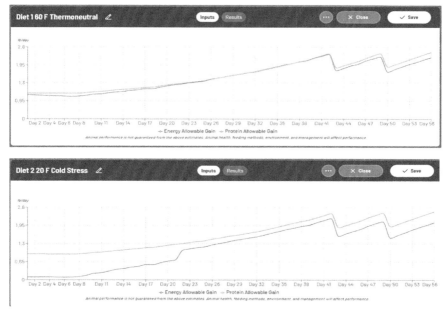

Fig. 4. Energy allowable gain (EAG) and protein allowable gain (PAG) results for comparison of calf growth performance between thermoneutral (60° F) and cold stress conditions (20° F) utilizing the Milk Specialties Global Calf Growth Model (https://toolkit.milkspecialties.com/).

EXAMPLE APPLICATION

As mentioned in the Introduction, one potential application of calf growth modeling programs is the evaluation of the impact of cold stress on the overall gain during the preweaning phase. The Milk Specialties Global Calf Growth Model will be used to demonstrate this application.

Two diets were created and the inputs are shown in **Fig. 3**. An MR 24 to 20 (24% CP – 20% Fat) was used as the liquid feed ingredient and a Calf Starter 18% (18% CP) was used as the dry feed ingredient. The feeding rates of the ingredients remained the same between the 2 diets. Calf inputs were also the same between the 2 diets, with the only difference being the temperature inputs. The thermoneutral diet temperature input was set to 60° F (15.6° C) and the cold stress diet temperature input was set to 20° F (−6.7° C).

The results of the modeling analysis are displayed in **Fig. 4**. Energy allowable gain (EAG) and protein allowable gain (PAG) are represented graphically for each day of the feeding period. Cold stress diverts energy resources from the diet toward meeting the increased maintenance energy needs of the calf, resulting in less energy available for gain. This is particularly noticeable during the first 3 weeks of the feeding period.

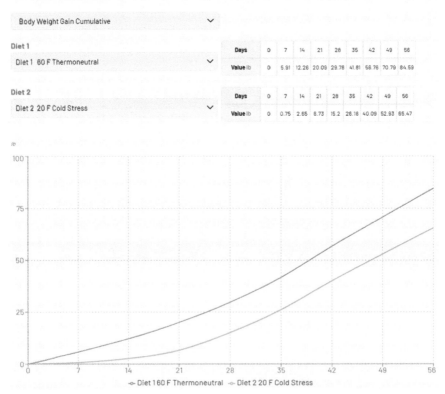

Compare Diets

| Body Weight Gain Cumulative | ⌄ |

Diet 1

Diet 1 60 F Thermoneutral ⌄

Days	0	7	14	21	28	35	42	49	56
Value lb	0	5.91	12.26	20.09	29.78	41.81	58.76	70.79	84.59

Diet 2

Diet 2 20 F Cold Stress ⌄

Days	0	7	14	21	28	35	42	49	56
Value lb	0	0.75	2.65	8.73	15.2	26.16	40.09	52.93	65.47

-o- Diet 1 60 F Thermoneutral -o- Diet 2 20 F Cold Stress

Fig. 5. Comparison of body weight gain between thermoneutral (60° F) and cold stress conditions (20° F) using Compare function within the Milk Specialties Global Calf Growth Model (https://toolkit.milkspecialties.com/).

The compare function within the Milk Specialties Calf Growth Model allows one to select and compare a result parameter between any 2 diets (**Fig. 5**). In this example application, cold stress resulted in a decrease of body weight gain of approximately 19 lb when compared with thermoneutral conditions. In a real-world situation, there are going to be daily fluctuations in the ambient temperature. Nonetheless, this example underscores the impact that cold stress can have on calf performance and although the predicted actual body weight gains may not exactly mirror real-world situations, the relative differences seen in body weight gain is enough to warrant a modification in the feeding program to provide more energy in the face of cold stress.

SUMMARY

The development of modeling concepts with the 2001 NRC[5] represented a big step toward understanding and applying the underlying mechanisms associated with young calf growth. Refinement of the modeling equations progressed with a series of well-designed detailed research studies in the early 2000s looking at the impact of varying levels of protein and energy on body composition and overall gain. Factors such as breed and environmental stressors impact calf growth. Investigation into delivering the proper amounts of energy and protein through the liquid and dry feeds to optimize growth needs to continue as well as further defining the most effective means to transition from the nonruminant to ruminant phase while minimizing postweaning lag.

As calves of superior genetic merit continue to be identified, the management and nutrition practices used to commercially raise dairy calves, either as replacements for the dairy herd or for meat, will require an ongoing refinement and utilization of tools to optimize calf growth. Calf growth modeling, not only during the preweaning phase but throughout the entire growth period, will be one such tool that can be used in this age of continuous improvement.

DISCLOSURE

Rich Larson has worked part-time and on a consulting basis for Milk Specialties Global, a manufacturer of rumen bypass fat supplements and milk replacers for the dairy industry.

REFERENCES

1. Drackley JK. Calf nutrition from birth to breeding. Vet Clin Food Anim 2008;24: 55–86.
2. Hu W, Hill TM, Dennis TS, et al. Effects of milk replacer feeding rates on growth performance of Holstein dairy calves to 4 months of age, evaluated via a meta-analytical approach. J Dairy Sci 2020;013:2217–32.
3. Soberon F, Raffrenato E, Everett RW, et al. Preweaning milk replacer intake and effects on long-term productivity of dairy calves. J Dairy Sci 2012;95:783–93.
4. von Keyserlingk MAG, Wolf F, Hotzel M, et al. Effects of continuous versus periodic milk availability on behavior and performance of dairy calves. J Dairy Sci 2006;89:2126–31.
5. National Research Council. Nutrient requirements of dairy cattle. 7th edition. Washington, DC: National Academy Press; 2001.
6. Diaz MC, Van Amburgh ME, Smith JM, et al. Composition of growth of Holstein calves fed milk replacer from birth to 105-kilogram body weight. J Dairy Sci 2001;84:830–42.

7. Tikofsky JN, Van Amburgh ME, Ross DA. Effect of varying carbohydrate and fat content of milk replacer on body composition of Holstein bull calves. J Anim Sci 2001;79:2260–7.

8. Blome RM, Drackley JK, McKeith FK, et al. Growth, nutrient utilization, and body composition of dairy calves fed milk replacers containing dierent amounts of protein. J Anim Sci 2003;81:1641–55.

9. Bartlett KS, McKeith FK, VandeHaar MJ, et al. Growth and body composition of dairy calves fed milk replacers containing dierent amounts of protein at two feeding rates. J Anim Sci 2006;84:1454–67.

10. Van Amburgh ME, Drackley JK. 2005. Current perspectives on the energy and protein requirements of the pre-weaned calf. In: Garnsworthy PC, editor. Calf and heifer rearing. Nottingham, UK: Nottingham University Press; 2005. p. 67–82.

11. Calves in AMTS.Cattle.Pro. agricultural modeling & training systems web site. Available at: https://agmodelsystems.com/calves-in-amts-cattle-pro/. May 2021.

12. Wiedmeier RD, Young AJ, Hammon DS. Frequent changing and rinsing of drinking water buckets improved performance of hutch-reared Holstein calves. Bovine Pract 2006;40:1–6.

13. Place NT, Heinrichs AJ, Erb HN. The effects of disease, management, and nutrition on average daily gain of dairy heifers from birth to four months. J Dairy Sci 1998;81:1004–9.

14. Chester-Jones H, Heins BJ, Ziegler D, et al. Relationships between early-life growth, intake, and birth season with first-lactation performance of Holstein dairy cows. J Dairy Sci 2016;100:3697–704.

15. Bascom SA, James RE, McGilliard ML, et al. Influence of dietary fat and protein on body composition of jersey. Bull Calves J Dairy Sci 2007;90:5600–9.

16. Khan MA, Weary DM, von Keyserlingk MAG. Invited review: effects of milk ration on solid feed intake, weaning, and performance in dairy heifers. J Dairy Sci 2011; 94:1071–81.

17. Raeth-Knight M, Chester-Jones H, Hayes S, et al. Impact of conventional or intensive milk replacer programs on Holstein heifer performance through six months of age and during first lactation. J Dairy Sci 2009;92:799–809.

18. Gelsinger SL, Heinrichs AJ, Jones CM. A meta-analysis of the effects of pre-weaned calf nutrition and growth on first-lactation performance. J Dairy Sci 2016;99:6206–14.

19. Calf Note #58. Predicting calf starter intake in Holstein calves. Calf Notes website. 1999. Available at: https://calfnotes.com/pdffiles/CN058.pdf. May 2021.

Commercial Dairy Calf Management
Impact on Performance and Health

James Grothe, BS[a],*, R.M. Thornsberry, DVM, MBA[b]

KEYWORDS

- Commercial dairy calves • Stress • Transition • Grouping • Management

KEY POINTS

- Calves in transition from a milk replacer-based diet to a grain-based diet exhibit stress, demonstrated by increased serum cortisol and α_1-acid glycoprotein levels at specific points in their lives that may influence subsequent health and performance.
- Using a "three C's" client education tool to influence calf management on the farm is an acceptable method for nutritionists and practicing veterinarians to influence calf managers' decision-making process:
  - Comfort—Consider calf comfort for every aspect of calf behavior and environment.
  - Consistency—Keeping life changes and interruptions to a minimum will yield better performance.
  - Calories—Formulating calf diets to be optimally energy dense will impact calf performance and health.

INTRODUCTION

Dairy calf production has changed over the last 30+ years, primarily due to increased population density in facility. One of the most difficult stages of production is weaning and the subsequent grouping of calves. This is a very critical life stage, as it has a direct effect on later production of both milk and meat. Understanding and reducing the intensity of sudden change in behavior and environment can reduce stress, which will improve performance.

Statistical testing in trials reviewed was not always similar. The authors of this article have listed those values in the text considered important to interpretation of outcomes, with trends being $P \leq .10$, significant being $P \leq .05$, and highly significant declared at $P \leq .01$. The significance values are reported as presented in the articles reviewed. All photographs are the property of R.M. Thornsberry D.V.M. and are reproduced with permission.

[a] Agriculture Education, University of Minnesota; [b] Mid America Veterinary Consulting, PO Box 818, Richland, MO 65556, USA
* Corresponding author. 2905 Highway 61N, Muscatine, IA 52761
E-mail address: james.grothe@kentww.com

Vet Clin Food Anim 38 (2022) 63–75
https://doi.org/10.1016/j.cvfa.2021.11.005
0749-0720/22/© 2021 Elsevier Inc. All rights reserved.

THE "THREE C'S" OF COMMERCIAL DAIRY CALF PRODUCTION

Comfort begins with good clean dry, deep bedding. The bedding material should be wheat or barley straw, not corn stover (stalks), bean fodder, or grass hay. Straw provides a better nesting score compared with other bedding types. Research conducted by the University of Wisconsin demonstrated that deep bedding in straw reduced the incidence of bovine respiratory disease (BRD) (P<.002).[1] The hollow stem of straw captures air and provides an insulation impact for calves. Although this research evaluated bedding types and amounts in winter months, a University of Arkansas study evaluated bedding materials for Holstein replacement dairy heifers raised in summer and fall.[2] These researchers evaluated granite fines, sand, rice hulls, long wheat straw, and wood shavings. Growth rates and feed efficiency were not different among bedding materials from day 1 through 42. The authors noted this lack of significant difference may have been influenced by the milk replacer only providing 14.4% crude fat, possibly confounding growth and performance.[3] Calves bedded on granite fines and sand had higher rates of antibiotic treatments (P<.05) during the first 2 weeks on milk replacer. Wheat straw bedded calves had the lowest recorded scours scores, based on the number of days calves exhibited a liquid stool. Observations on calf cleanliness varied among bedding types (P<.05). Calves bedded with granite fines and sand were the dirtiest 2 groups. The calves with the wettest hair coats were bedded on sand. Although bedding types did not significantly impact final 42-day performance parameters, they did impact scours score and treatment frequency. Calf comfort is important.

This Arkansas study also measured bedding type effect on serum cortisol concentration. Serum cortisol levels were highest on day 1, but did not differ among bedding types. Higgenbotham and Stull (1997)[4] observed similar serum cortisol levels in their calf research, recording the highest levels at day 1, which gradually decreased through week 3. Serum α_1-acid glycoprotein (AGP) was also measured. AGP was highest on day 1 and gradually decreased throughout the 42-day study. Bedding types had no impact on AGP numbers. Serum APG level is recognized as a predictor of death in aging humans[5] and of stress in calves.[6]

Self-grooming is normal calf behavior for calves of all ages. A Chinese study documented individually housed calves self-groomed 40.7 minutes per day and paired housed calves self-groomed 20.6 minutes per day ($\pm$4.10 minutes per day; $P = .02$).[7] Cameras with infrared technology posted above each calf pen were used to record self-grooming behavior data points. Self-grooming time decreased when calves were grouped after weaning, indicating the increased time devoted to self-grooming activity in individually housed calves could be an indicator of mental calf stress. The Arkansas bedding materials study recorded increased self-grooming for calves housed on rice hulls and sand compared with long wheat straw. As calves self-groom, they potentially recycle intestinal pathogens from their own feces and pen mate's feces adhered to their hair coats. Clean, absorbent bedding is important to keeping calves clean and dry. A 2018 study[8] demonstrated that sick calves (those experimentally infected with *Mannheimia haemolytica*) exhibited reduced self-grooming times, feeding activity, and social interaction—spending more time lying down, especially in lateral recumbency, compared with their healthy pen mates. The authors suggested that calf managers should observe calves closely, as behavioral changes may be indicative of early onset of BRD. One- to 3-month-old calves appear to be most susceptible to BRD.[9]

Although results in feedlot cattle cannot be directly applied to raising commercial dairy calves up to 400 pounds (181.8 KG), performance improvement findings should apply as dairy calves increase in age and weight. A North Dakota State University study[10] reported improved daily gain and total weight gain for feedlot steers double-bedded with wheat straw compared with calves lightly bedded with wheat straw or not bedded ($P<.05$). Steers receiving no bedding exhibited an average daily gain (ADG) of 2.83 lb/d (1.29 kg/d). Lightly bedded steers had an ADG of 3.69 lb/d (1.67 kg/d), whereas double-bedded steers gained 3.53 lb/d (1.60 kg/d). Gain per feed intake improved ($P = .06$) in one study period and overall for both bedded groups ($P = .06$). In a second experiment, the authors examined the impact of various bedding materials. Calves bedded on wheat straw gained fastest ($P<.01$), followed by soybean fodder, corn stover (stalks), and calves with no bedding, for pens scraped twice weekly. Wheat straw bedding is the time-honored bedding material, especially so for younger calves. Other research agrees with the finding of this study, but results from these studies were not as dramatic.[11–13] The results from these 4 studies demonstrate the economic impact of calf comfort.

There are many factors that influence the incidence and severity of respiratory disease in dairy calves. Philip J. Griebel, DVM, Vaccine and Infectious Disease Organization, University of Saskatchewan, in a recent presentation, presented data to support that a combination of psychological and nutritional stressors associated with abrupt weaning significantly enhance fatal BRD. Stressors appear to have a direct effect on the amplitude of antiviral responses. Surprisingly, stressors enhanced, rather than inhibited, innate immune responses to infection with infectious bovine rhinotracheitis virus, actually exaggerating the immune system's normal responses to infection.[14]

At the 2009 American Association of Bovine Practitioners annual convention, Griebel said functional genomic analyses suggest antiviral responses were linked to an increased capacity to respond to gram-negative bacterial respiratory infections through increased expression of TLR4 (toll-like receptor 4) and CD14 (receptor sites on the surface of macrophages). As these specific receptors are activated, the immune system in effect overreacts to the presence of certain types of pneumonia-causing bacteria, increasing the severity of disease expression. The end result is increased morbidity—disease case expression in a given population—and an increased incidence of mortality.[15,16]

As receptors respond to substances produced by infecting bacteria that have succumbed to immune system responses, the dead bacteria release chemical substances into the surrounding lung tissue. In response to these chemicals, the immune system rushes in white blood cells, causing infiltration of cellular components of the immune system, which subsequently damages the lung tissue, causing swelling and fluid accumulation. Veterinarians will often comment, while performing a postmortem examination on calves that have died of complications resulting from pneumonia, that the lungs look, and actually feel like, liver tissue rather than lung tissue. The lung tissue has become so heavy with fluid, serum, and cellular material that it literally takes on the appearance of liver tissue, both visually and tactilely. This tissue can no longer exchange oxygen from the inhaled air, nor can it release carbon dioxide with the exhaled air, and if enough lung tissue is damaged or enough bacterial toxins are absorbed, the calf dies. This immunologic knowledge provides evidence for a novel mechanism by which stress may enhance the risk of fatal BRD.[14] In addition, modulation of TLR4 expression during viral infection may be of relevance for both gram-negative and gram-positive bacterial infections. Both types of bacteria are common causes of bacterial pneumonia and bacterial mastitis. Stress, and particularly, stacking stressors, should be avoided at all costs, and the knowledge of how stress influences disease expression in calves should be used as a management tool by modern dairy calf raisers.

Although it is possible to have sudden onset of pneumonia and respiratory disease expression that is primarily caused by a bacterial infection in individual calves, the usual scenario for a severe respiratory outbreak in a group of calves involves a primary infection by a bovine respiratory virus, followed by an induced secondary bacterial pneumonia. This knowledge makes it imperative that calves be vaccinated against the most common respiratory viral causes of BRD early in life so immunity is established long before a potential stress or stressor event is to occur.

This finding also supports the gradual weaning of wet calves. An acceptable gradual weaning can be accomplished by dropping one feeding for 3 days, then feeding every other day for 3 days, and weaning the calves off milk on day 7.[17] It is recommended to leave calves in their original housing for a period of 2 weeks after weaning. This weaning process ties up housing for a 3-week period, but allows the calf to begin the process of consuming enough starter feed to survive before placing the calves in group housing where they must compete with one another for intake. It is generally recommended by dairy calf nutritionists that calves should be consuming 3 pounds (1.36 kg) of a good quality starter feed before weaning.[18] Although earlier and earlier weaning is becoming the norm in modern calf raising facilities, most practicing food animal veterinarians would caution producers on weaning too early, as adding the stress of weaning at too early an age, before the immune system becoming well established with a proper response to vaccinations, should be a consideration. Establishing immunity takes time. It is important that a proper immune response with both a sensitized cell-mediated immune system and circulating antibodies be established before weaning.

Stacking stressors should be avoided at all costs. Do not perform any management practice at weaning except weaning. Do not castrate, dehorn, vaccinate, change feed, move to different housing, or group calves at weaning. Allow the calf to accustom itself to the stress of weaning, and allow the stressful event to abate before moving to new housing or grouping with other calves. It is generally recognized that 2 weeks' time is required to deal with one stressor, much less several stacked on top of one another.[19] By following a process of gradual weaning, calves are much more capable of handling the stress of being removed from a liquid diet. Gradual weaning will also promote proper and stepped increases in starter feed intake.[20] Can calves be abruptly weaned by simply not feeding the milk or milk replacer 1 day? Yes, but there may be consequences of an increased incidence of respiratory diseases, and a slump in performance. There are data generated to support gradual weaning of wet calves off milk or milk replacer.[20] Producers should note that dairy calves increase water intake the day of weaning by about 30%.[21] Provide ample clean, fresh water at the time of weaning. Water intake directly influences dry feed intake.[22]

Grouping calves after the process of weaning, and the size of the group, contributed to the severity and the incidence of respiratory disease.[23] It was determined that calves should be grouped in no larger groups than 9 head, with better performance achieved in the smaller groups, 6 head per group pen. A study performed in Norway determined that calves housed together before 1 month of age had a greater risk of dying compared with calves housed individually.[24] Although there is debate about how many square feet there should be in a group pen, it is generally recognized that at least 40 to 50 square feet (12.19 by 15.24 m^2) per calf is needed for optimal performance[25] (**Fig. 1**). A pen of 6 weaned calves would require a pen size that is at least 10 feet (3.05 m) wide by 30 feet (9.15 m) in length, and a 10 head pen would require a pen that is 20 feet (6.09 m) by 30 feet (9.15 m) (**Fig. 2**). It has been determined that if enough space is not allowed for grouped calves, there is a greater risk of developing infectious diarrhea.[26]

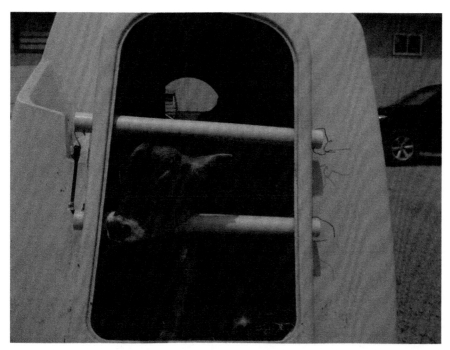

Fig. 1. Calves need more room than the space in a calf hutch. A hutch is fine for the first few days of life, as is the case for this newborn Jersey calf, but after a few days, calves need some exercise room.

Proper shelter is important to keep rain, snow, and sleet off calves, but it is vital that the bedded area be kept dry and clean. Bacteria and parasites need moisture to reproduce and complete their life cycle. Although deep bedding may not be required for calves grouped together after weaning, the bedding must be sufficient to maintain a dry clean environment. Frequent bedding may be necessary, particularly during times of wet weather (**Fig. 3**). Calves self-groom and socially groom throughout each day.[7] If manure and filth have accumulated on their legs, hips, and sides from lying in wet filthy bedding, the calves will simply recycle and reinfect themselves with what they lick off their hair coats while grooming (**Fig. 4**). Keep the bedding intervals close enough to secure a clean dry environment in the sheltering areas, as it may influence the incidence of intestinal disease. The shelter should be open enough to allow moisture to evaporate and to prevent poor ventilation conditions.[1]

Grouping calves after weaning is a stressful event. Cattle, like all domestic species, establish a pecking order within the group. Calves that were raised individually are not accustomed to competing with other calves for feed, space, or water. Make sure there is enough shelter for all calves in the group to comfortably lie down under the shelter, and make sure there is enough bunk space for all calves to comfortably eat at the same time. Bunk space is important at any stage of development, but especially so after weaning. Calves are social animals and desire to eat at the same time. As most calves at this point in management are limited to be fed 2.5 to 3% of their body weight in energy-dense feed, it is essential that all calves can consume their proper proportions at the same time. Water should be easy to access, and it must

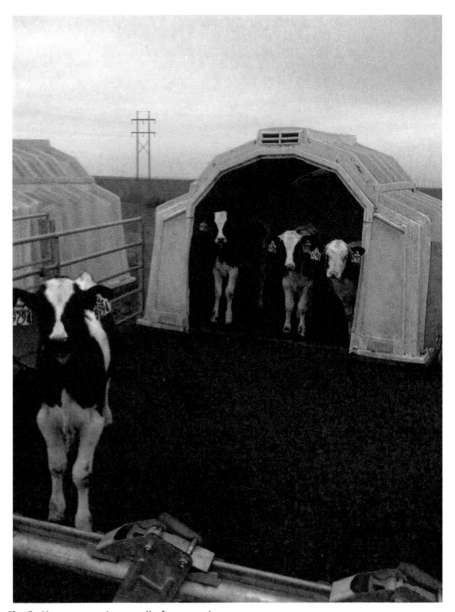

Fig. 2. Keep group sizes small after weaning.

be kept clean and fresh. Make sure the waterer is not too high for a calf to reach, and not so low as to become contaminated with feces. Group housing begins the process of socialization among calves, and is considered a major animal welfare issue for today's animal husbandry practices.[27]

With a good vaccination protocol to establish immunity against common bovine respiratory pathogens, and armed with the knowledge that stress increases both the incidence and severity of respiratory disease, the calf manager can take the appropriate

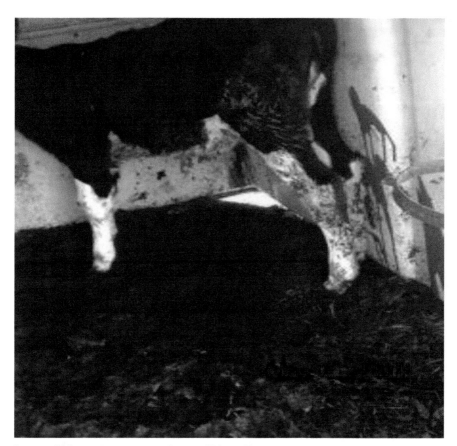

Fig. 3. A filthy environment produces a filthy calf!

steps to insure the best possible environment for weaning and grouping calves after the milk or milk replacer feeding period of production. A little attention to detail will pay off in healthy replacement heifers with potential for future milk production ability. It will prepare dairy beef calves for future production efficiencies in the feedlot.

Comfort is important for accessibility to clean, fresh water and feed. The height of bunks and water sources should not be too tall. When a calf eats or drinks, there should not be more than 24 inches (61 cm) total from where the calf stands to the bottom of the bunk. To check this, take a tape measure and hold one end on the ground where the calf stands and run the tape up to the edge of the bunk and then back down to where the calf consumes the feed or water, the bottom of the feed bunk or trough. That measurement needs to be 24 inches or less (61 cm) and applies to the waterer as well. Bunks or troughs should be designed to keep feed fresh and free from contamination. Fresh feed is important to stimulate proper daily feed intake. Feed bunks should be off the ground and preferably polylined (**Fig. 5**). Polylined bunks are easy to clean and will keep the feed fresh and palatable.

Feed bunks should be cleaned of foreign material and fines weekly (**Fig. 6**). Feeding twice daily for the first 28 days in a transition facility will increase daily feed intake, as it mimics starter feed provision practices the calves were accustomed to before

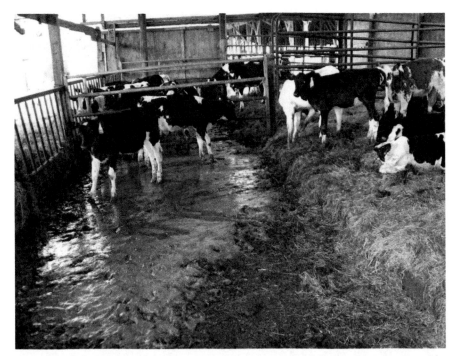

Fig. 4. Weaned calves improperly managed are quite typical for the weaning transition phase of dairy calf production. Feces removal and bedding management are basic animal husbandry practices that must be observed to prevent the development of a coccidiosis or *Nematodirus spp.* outbreak.

grouping. This provides the human interaction the calves crave and stimulates feed intake. Feeding twice daily keeps the feed fresher, which also improves feed intake. This will insure the calves are checked twice a day to be able to diagnose unhealthy calves in a timelier fashion. Waterers need to be checked daily for foreign material and cleaned weekly (**Fig. 7**). It takes 4 pounds (1.82 kg) of water to digest 1 pound (0.454 kg) of feed.[22]

Consistency is important to commercial calf management. Transition is a stressful event, but keeping management and feeding times similar to the times used in the milk replacer feeding time of production, will provide the calf a familiar routine. Use the same starter feed in the transition facility for the first 2 weeks, and transition to the grower diets slowly. It takes about 2 weeks for calves to adjust to feed and environmental changes.[19] Limit the distance hauled or time required to move calves from the calf raising facility to the transition facility. Refrain from any planned veterinary intervention events a week before or 2 to 3 weeks after grouping. It is critical to keep stress manageable at transition. Do not vaccinate, castrate, debud, or dehorn until 2 to 3 weeks after grouping. Group calves as to maturity and weight to keep socialization stress to a minimum. Do not wean too early. Calves need some maturity to compete in a group housing transition facility. Calves should be 9 to 10 weeks old when they are grouped. Once calves are grouped, keep them together until 350 to 400 pounds (159–182 kg) to reduce the comingling and socialization stress.

It is best to read bunks at a similar time every day to determine when to increase intake. A good policy is when the bunk is empty for 3 straight mornings; increase

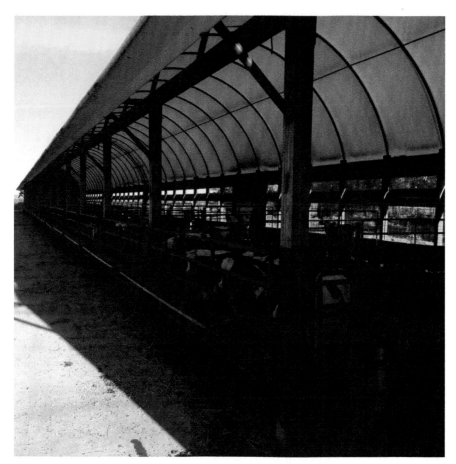

Fig. 5. A hoop structure transition facility in South Dakota. Note polylined protected feed bunks. Waterers inside each 10 head pens do result in water contamination of the pens on hot days when calves flutter the water out of the waterers into the bedded pen areas.

the intake to a maximum of 1 pound (0.454 kg) per head per day. Producers should target feed intakes to be at 3% to 4% of body weight.

A calorie is a term used in common literature that producers can understand as energy provision. Feed manufacturing and ingredients are both important to daily feed intake for calves. The starter feed will be a high-quality feed with a high net energy for gain. Producers can be tempted to reduce the cost of the transition and grower feed. A total mixed ration (TMR) containing wet feed sources, such as corn silage or haylage of some sort, is not a good option for transitioning calves. Wet feeds are 60% moisture by weight. Newly weaned calves do not have the rumen capacity to consume enough wet forage-based TMR to meet their daily energy intake requirements. Newly weaned calves should be fed the same feed they received at the calf facility for at least the first 2 to 3 weeks in a transition facility. A recommended grower transition diet would contain whole corn, pellet for protein, and macronutrient and micronutrient supplementation, with 10% to 15% oats. Using something to reduce the dust is recommended to increase intake, such as corn or soy oil, or molasses.

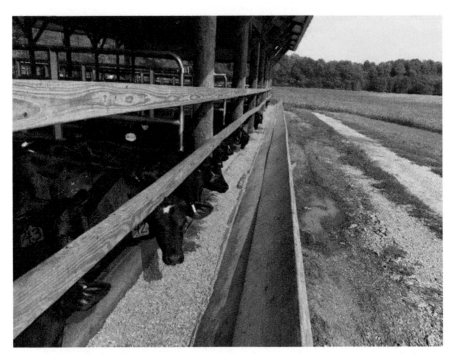

Fig. 6. Illinois transition facility with clean wooden feed troughs. Waterers are at the back of each 10 head pen.

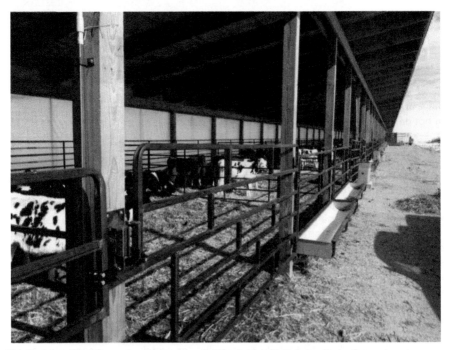

Fig. 7. A modified open front transition facility in South Dakota. Note the waterers are on the outside of each 10 head pen. This keeps water contamination of the pens on hot days to a minimum.

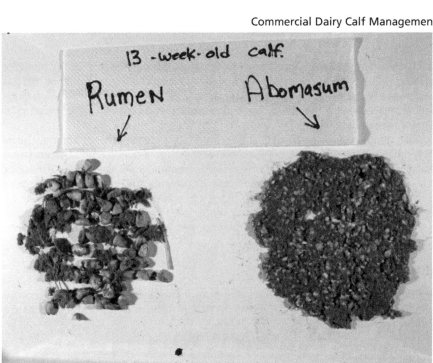

Fig. 8. Whole corn stimulates rumen development. Chewing during eructation and rumination reduces particle size.

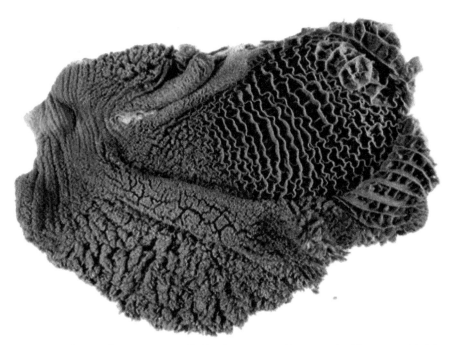

Fig. 9. Note the excellent rumen papilli development in this 13-week-old commercial dairy calf rumen. Whole corn diets reduce the cost of processing and provide a nutritional stimulus for rumen development.[29]

Intake should be about 3% of body weight. It is recommended to start transition calves on a 18% crude protein diet, gradually reducing the crude protein to 16% as the calves approach 400 pounds (182 kg). The use of high fiber commodity feed ingredients can greatly limit the energy content of a calf diet. Energy intake is important to immune system function.[28]

Whole corn provides good palatability and is an excellent energy source. Calves chew much of the corn during consumption and rechew it during eructation and rumination, which allows for excellent particle size for rumen fermentation (**Fig. 8**). Feeding any type of forage is not recommended until 300 pounds (159 kg). Good quality grass hay fed at 1 to 2 pounds (0.454–0.908 kg) per day is adequate at that time. Rumen capacity is limited in calves under 300 to 400 pounds (159–182 kg). Free choice access to forage will limit grain intake simply due to rumen fill, and performance will diminish due to poor rumen development (**Fig. 9**).

SUMMARY

Implementing management practices that provide the "three C's" of comfort, consistency, and calories will improve health and performance in weaned and transitioning commercial dairy calves.

DISCLOSURE

The authors have nothing to disclose.

REFERENCES

1. Largo A, McQuirk SM, Bennett TB, et al. Calf respiratory disease and pen micro-environments in naturally ventilated calf barns in winter. J Dairy Sci 2006;89: 4014–25.
2. Panivivat R, Kegley EB, Pennington JA, et al. Growth performance and health in dairy calves bedded with different types of materials. J Dairy Sci 2004;87: 3736–45.
3. Scibilia LS, Muller SL, Kensinger RS, et al. Effect of environmental temperature and dietary fat on growth and physiological responses of new-born calves. J Dairy Sci 1987;70:1426–33.
4. Higginbotham GE, Stull CL. Performance and health of dairy calves using different types of commercial housing. Prof Anim Sci 1997;13:18–23.
5. Henry OF, Blacher J, Verdavaine J, et al. Alpha 1-acid glycoprotein is an independent predictor of in-hospital death in the elderly. Aging 2003;32(1):37–42.
6. Itoh H, Tamura K, Izumi M, et al. Characterization of serum $alpha_1$-acid glycoprotein in fetal and newborn calves during development. Am J Vet Res 1993;54: 591–5.
7. Liu S, Ma J, Li J, et al. Effects of pair versus individual housing on performance, health, and behavior of dairy calves. Animal 2020;10:50.
8. Hixson CL, Krawczel PD, Caldwell JM, et al. Behavioral changes in group-housed dairy calves infected with *Mannheimia haemolytica*. J Dairy Sci 2018;101: 10351–60.
9. Bryson D. Calf pneumonia. Vet Clin North Am Food Anim Pract 1985;2:237–57.
10. Anderson VL, Wiederholt RJ, Schoonmaker JP. Effects of bedding feedlot cattle during the winter on performance, carcass quality, and nutrients in manure. Carrington Res Extension Cent Beef Rep 2006;29:28–36.

11. Anderson VL, Aberle E, Swenson L. Effects of bedding on winter performance of feedlot cattle and nutrient conservation in composted manure. J Anim Sci 2005; 83(Supple 1). Abstract (2).
12. Birkelo, C.P. and J. Lounsbery. 1992. Effect of straw and newspaper bedding on cold season feedlot performance in two housing systems. South Dakota Beef Report p.42-45.
13. Stanton, T.L., and D. N. Schutz. 1996. Effect of bedding on finishing cattle performance and carcass characteristics. Colorado State Univ., Agric. Exp. Sta. J. Ser. No. 1-5 606.
14. Hodgson PD, Aich P, Manuja A, et al. Effect of stress on viral-bacterial synergy in bovine respiratory disease: novel mechanisms to regulate inflammation. Comp Funct Genomics 2005;6:244–50.
15. Aick P, Potter AA, Griebel PJ. Modern approaches to understanding stress and disease susceptibility: A review with special emphasis on respiratory disease. Int J Gen Med 2009;2:19–32.
16. Van Der Fels-Klerx HJ, Martin SW, Nielen M, et al. Effects on productivity and risk factors of bovine respiratory disease in dairy heifers: A review for the Netherlands. Neth J Agric Sci 2002;50:27–45.
17. Khan MA, Lee HJ, Lee WS, et al. Pre- and postweaning performance of Holstein female calves fed milk through step-down and conventional methods. J Dairy Sci 2007;90:876–85.
18. Khan MA, Bach A, Weary DM, et al. Invited review: Transitioning from milk to solid feed in dairy heifers. J Dairy Sci 2016;99:885–902.
19. Tomkins T, Jaster EH. Preruminant calf nutrition. Vet Clin North Amer Food Anim Pract. 1991;7:557.
20. Sweeney BC, Rushen J, Weary DM, et al. Duration of weaning, starter intake, and weight gain of dairy calves fed large amounts of milk. J Dairy Sci 2010;93(1): 148–52.
21. Overvest MA, Crossley RE, Miller-Cushon EK, et al. Social housing influences the behavior and feed intake of dairy calves during weaning. J Dairy Sci 2018;101: 8123–34.
22. Kertz AF, Reutzel LF, Mahoney JH. Ad libitum water intake by neonatal calves and its relationship to calf starter intake, weight gain, feces score, and season. J Dairy Sci 1984;67:2964–9.
23. Lundborg GK, Svensson EC, Oltenacu PA. Herd-level risk factors for infectious diseases in Swedish dairy calves aged 0-90 days. Prev Vet Med 2005;68:123–43.
24. Gulliksen SM, Lie KI, Loken T, et al. Calf mortality in Norwegian dairy herds. J Dairy Sci 2009b;92:2782–95.
25. Penn State University, Management of Dairy Heifers, Extension Circular 385.
26. Bendali F, Sanaa M, Bichet H, et al. Risk factors associated with diarrhoea in newborn calves. Vet Res 1999;30:509–22.
27. Gulliksen SM, Jor E, Lie KI, et al. Respiratory infections in Norwegian dairy calves. J Dairy Sci 2009a;92:5139–46.
28. Pollock JM, Rowan TG, Dixon JB, et al. Alteration of cellular immune responses by nutrition and weaning in calves. Res Vet Sci 1993;55:298–306.
29. Zitman R, Voigt J, Schonhusen U, et al. Influence of dietary concentrate to forage ratio on the development of rumen mucosa in calves. Arch Tierernahr 1998;51(4): 279–91.

Preparing Male Dairy Calves for the Veal and Dairy Beef Industry

David Renaud, DVM, PhD[a],*, Bart Pardon, DVM, PhD[b]

KEYWORDS

- Bovine respiratory disease • Stress • Health management • Antimicrobial use
- Body weight

KEY POINTS

- The veal and dairy beef sectors are essential to the dairy industry to valorize excess male calves and represent a billion-dollar industry.
- Despite that mortality rates are similar to the dairy industry, to maintain healthy calves the veal and dairy beef industry heavily rely on antimicrobial use, resulting in high levels of antimicrobial resistance.
- Calves with reduced morbidity risk and better production can be identified based on arrival parameters of which body weight and immunoglobulin concentration are most informative.
- At the dairy herds of origin, key factors to improve veal and dairy calf health are assuring an adequate body weight before transport (>50 kg (>110 lbs)), adequate transfer of passive immunity, and specific immunity by vaccination. The accumulation of stressors, in particular transport related, needs to be avoided or alleviated.
- At the veal and dairy beef herds, calves should be classified according to disease risk and receive appropriate arrival management, limiting antimicrobial use to high-risk animals.

INTRODUCTION

The veal and dairy beef sectors are important outlets for surplus calves from the dairy industry. Surplus calves are defined as calves that are not needed to produce milk, with the majority being male and the remainder comprising females that are not needed as replacement dairy animals.[1] In Canada and the United States, it is estimated that more than 5.2 million male dairy calves were produced by the dairy industry in 2020.[2,3] In the European Union (including the United Kingdom), about 11 million

[a] Department of Population Medicine, Ontario Veterinary College, University of Guelph, Guelph, Ontario, Canada; [b] Department of Internal Medicine, Reproduction and Population Medicine, Faculty of Veterinary Medicine, Ghent University, Salisburylaan 133, Merelbeke 9820, Belgium
* Corresponding author.
E-mail address: renaudd@uoguelph.ca

Vet Clin Food Anim 38 (2022) 77–92
https://doi.org/10.1016/j.cvfa.2021.11.006
0749-0720/22/© 2021 Elsevier Inc. All rights reserved.

male dairy calves were produced in 2020.[4] A meaningful number of female calves are also not needed as replacements within the dairy industry due to the increased use of sexed semen.[5] It is more difficult to place an exact number of surplus female calves, but it is estimated to be several million animals per year globally.

Traditionally in North America and Europe, most of the surplus dairy calves have entered the veal industry comprised of the milk-fed (also referred to as white veal or special fed) and grain-fed (also referred to as red, rose, or nonformula-fed) veal sectors.[6] Milk-fed veal is one of the more traditional forms of veal production whereby calves are fed a diet comprised of mainly high volumes of milk replacer with a small amount of forage. This sector is highly integrated whereby a small number of companies raise and slaughter most of the milk-fed veal calves. In contrast, next to large facilities in the EU, grain-fed veal production occurs more frequently on smaller, mostly privately owned farms whereby they are fed small volumes of milk replacer, are weaned, and transitioned onto a corn-based diet. A similarity between the 2 sectors is that both slaughter calves before 8 months of age. In Europe, veal production comprises approximately 14% of the total amount of bovine meat produced,[7] whereas, in Canada, veal comprises only 6% of bovine meat produced.[8]

Another important outlet for surplus dairy calves is the dairy-beef market.[9] Although not a new industry, the exponential increase in the use of beef semen in dairy cows with low genetic value has led to new market opportunities.[10] For example, in auction markets in Quebec, Canada the number of cross-bred calves has increased from 7% of calves going through auction in 2016 to more than 30% being cross-bred in 2020.[11] This increase in the number of available crossed-breed calves has led to a further increase in the dairy-beef market which starts the calves similar to the grain-fed veal industry, however, finishes the calves using a silage-based ration whereby calves are slaughtered around 18 to 24 months of age. This outlet likely will increase through time due to the declining veal market in North America but may also displace portions of the beef market for a variety of reasons including a lower environmental impact in raising cross-bred dairy calves than traditional beef.[12]

Regardless of the outlet proposed, the surplus male dairy calves are a huge reputational issue for the dairy industry worldwide because of public concern for animal welfare.[1,13,14] The transportation of animals at a young age and crowding in facilities without outdoor access, preventing the animals from expressing natural behavior, are the key criticisms. On the other hand, "solutions" like immediate euthanasia after birth or slaughter at a very young age ('bobby calves') are very unlikely to find public support in North America and the EU. Clearly, to avoid drastic but unsuccessful long-term investments in alternative systems as happened in the poultry industry, the dairy industry urgently needs to consult consumers and other stakeholders to develop a sustainable model for their surplus calves in the future to have the social license to produce.

Part of the short-term solution likely lies in improving the current model combined with more transparency on morbidity, mortality, antimicrobial use, and welfare. In this narrative review, the authors provide an overview of possible management factors that can be conducted at the farm of origin and at the veal/dairy beef facility to reduce disease burden and the associated antimicrobial use and welfare issues.

Major Challenges in Veal and Dairy Beef Sectors

Historically, restrictive housing and diets consisting solely of milk replacer were the major public criticisms of veal production.[15] However, in Europe and parts of North America, the implementation of laws and codes of practice has changed these components of the sector substantially. Nevertheless, nonnutritive behavior and other signs of insufficient animal welfare are still frequent in veal production which requires further refinement.[16]

A major challenge within the current structure of the veal and dairy beef sectors is the high levels of antimicrobial use.[17] Of the cattle industries, the veal sector remains the highest user of antimicrobials despite the use of laws and sector initiatives within the European Union.[18,19] In addition, of all cattle sectors, the highest levels of antimicrobial resistance in commensal bacteria and pathogens are found within the veal industry.[20,21] Important zoonotic agents like livestock-associated methicillin-resistant *Staphylococcus aureus* (LA-MRSA) and extended beta-lactamase (ESBL) harboring *Enterobacteriaceae* are also highly prevalent in the veal calf sector.[22,23] To safeguard the efficacy of antimicrobials, an urgent reduction of antimicrobial consumption in food animals is needed.[24]

One of the main factors driving the use of antimicrobials is the exceptionally high disease burden within the veal industry.[18] A reason for this level of disease is that calves originate from a multitude of herds (e.g., about 1.3 calves/herd of origin in Belgium[25]), resulting in an almost 100% chance of bringing every infectious disease possible into the veal or dairy beef farm. The main disease within the veal sector is a respiratory disease which accounts for more than 60% of antimicrobial use.[17] Next to the seasonal viruses, the prevalence of *Mycoplasma bovis* is tremendously high with almost all veal operations infected in contrast to dairy farms, whereby depending on the country, 20% to 30% are infected.[26–28] In addition to pathogen exposure, male dairy calves are exposed to an accumulation of stressors which are inherent to the current production system. In **Fig. 1**, an overview of the stressors male dairy calves are exposed to in the first 3 to 4 weeks of their life is provided. The multitude, extent, and duration of these stressors induce chronic stress in the calves, which has negative effects on immune function and disease resilience.[29]

Where Do These Challenges Start?

Although the challenges outlined above seem difficult to overcome, there has been a large body of literature highlighting that many challenges related to the health status of

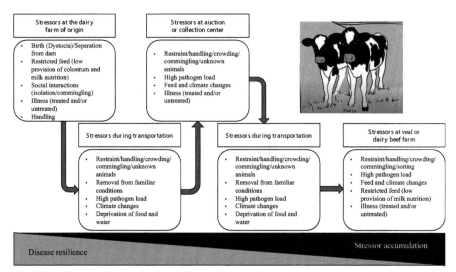

Fig. 1. An overview of the accumulation of the different repeated stressors in the current industry chain.

calves entering the veal and dairy beef industries. Many calves entering have been found to have noticeable health abnormalities with 13% to 23%, 3% to 20%, and 32% to 46% of calves either at the auction facility or on entry to a veal facility having diarrhea, an umbilical infection, and clinical dehydration, respectively.[30–36] A high number of calves also have low body weight and poor body condition.[34,35] As many of these parameters have been associated with future risk of morbidity and mortality as well as growth,[33,34,37] it is important to limit the entry of these "high-risk" calves into calf raising facilities.

Body weight at arrival to veal and dairy-beef facilities has been demonstrated to be the most important influencer of future mortality and morbidity risk as well as growth.[38] Specifically, higher levels of body weight are associated with a declining risk of reduced respiratory disease,[36,39] diarrhea,[36] morbidity,[33] and mortality,[34,36] especially in the first 21 days after arrival. In addition, calves that are heavier on arrival also have improved growth in the first 78 days after arrival[40] and over the entire production period.[37] Recently, an interaction of body weight with transport was demonstrated, whereby calves that were greater than 46 kg (>101 lbs) did not mount any acute phase response after a 2 h transport stress, whereas lightweight calves showed monocytosis and increased production of TNF-α and IL-17a.[41]

It is difficult to determine the ideal threshold for body weight at arrival; however, it could be speculated that it needs to be >50 kg (>110 lbs). Specifically, Brscic and others[39] identified that calves weighing greater than 51 kg (>112 lbs) at arrival had a lower risk of respiratory disease. In addition, others have found the optimal cutpoint for body weight at arrival being 46 kg (101 lbs) for predicting morbidity[40] and 44 to 47 kg (97–104 lbs) for mortality.[40,42] Although the sensitivity [62% for mortality[40,42]; 55% for morbidity[40]] and specificity [29% for mortality[40,42]; 46% for morbidity[40]] for predicting disease and death at these thresholds are limited, no other predictor that has been evaluated has more consistently predicted disease risk. Therefore, efforts are needed to maximize the body weight at arrival to improve calf health and growth.

Other clinical predictors have been associated with disease and mortality risk. Calves that are dehydrated at arrival, even mild cases (5%–6% dehydrated) have a higher risk of mortality and lower levels of growth.[34,42] Other studies showed that calves arriving with a depressed paralumbar fossa or sunken flank, umbilical infection, diarrhea, depressed attitude, or an induced cough have an increased mortality risk.[30,33,34,36] Whereas others found that calves with an umbilical infection and pyrexia have an increased risk of being treated for disease.[36] Therefore, ensuring calves are fit for sale before leaving the dairy farm will likely have a significant influence on disease risk and growth at calf raising facilities.

Despite the importance of having high levels of maternal immunoglobulins,[43] many calves arrive with failed transfer of passive immunity (FTPI), with a range of 12% to 43% of calves entering the veal or dairy-beef industry with FTPI.[32,36,44,45] It is not surprising that calves with FTPI are associated with a greater risk of morbidity and mortality. Specifically, calves with higher levels of total immunoglobulins, immunoglobulin G, and serum total protein had lower levels of mortality and disease.[40,42,45] Thresholds for the best prediction of mortality have been determined to be a serum IgG of 16.7 g/L to 19.85 g/L at arrival to veal facilities in calves approximately 1 week of age.[40,42] This supports that higher thresholds for passive immunity are needed[46] compared with the traditional threshold of 10 g/L. It is important to note that tests for FPTI based on total protein are not useful at greater than 9 days of age.[47] In Europe, male dairy calves need to be 14 days old before they can be transported, and at that age immunoglobulin levels less than 7.5 g/L have been associated with an increased BRD risk.[45] Although levels of maternal immunoglobulins are not the perfect predictor of mortality or morbidity, efforts to ensure that calves arrive with high levels will lead to better health and growth at calf raising facilities.[40]

Beyond levels of immunoglobulins in blood, other blood parameters have also been associated with disease risk. Lower cholesterol levels have been found in 2 studies to be associated with an increased risk of morbidity.[40,42] The reason for this association is unclear. However, it is speculated that calves that arrive at an older age, receive a higher volume of colostrum or nutrition before transit, and those that do not have a genetic haplotype deficiency will arrive with a higher level of cholesterol translating to a lower disease risk.[40] High levels of cortisol at arrival have also been found to be associated with disease risk. Specifically, Masmeijer and others[48] found that increasing levels of cortisol at arrival were associated with an increased risk for unresolving lung consolidation or chronic pneumonia. Calves are exposed to a multitude of stressors, but transport is likely key. Transport stress, which comprises loading, transporting, unloading, commingling, adverse weather conditions, and food and water deprivation, has been associated with reduced immune function in cattle.[49] Hence, minimizing stress before arrival is important in preventing disease, but clearly, the calves are exposed to multiple, accumulating stressors (see **Fig. 1**).[38]

Preconditioning Calves Destined to the Veal or Dairy-Beef Industry at the Dairy Farm of Origin

Preconditioning is the preparation of cattle at the farm of origin, so they cope better with stressors and pathogen exposures on the fattening farms.[50,51] In contrast to feedlot animals, there is little time for veal calves to be preconditioned given the young age at transport. Nevertheless, several measures can be taken at the dairy farm of origin to better prepare calves entering the veal or dairy-beef industries (**Table 1**).

As stated earlier, the most crucial measure is assuring an adequate body weight before departure from the dairy herd. A body weight of greater than 50 kg (>110 lbs) at a maximum age of 14 days is a reasonable target for male Holstein calves. Briefly, body weight is predominantly influenced by birth weight, nutritional plane and quality, and occurrence of disease. It is outside the scope of the present article to provide a complete overview of factors influencing birth weight of cattle. However, good management of maternal body condition scores contribute as calves from cows with higher body condition scores have lower birth weights and grow less rapid.[52] Similarly, supra-nutritional supplementation of dams with selenium resulted in higher calf birth weights and more efficient uptake of colostral IgG.[53] For economic reasons, the nutritional plane offered to male dairy calves is sometimes insufficient. This is an issue that can be easily tackled by the dairy industry if the correct motivational factors can be found. Any inflammatory process will mount an acute phase response (innate immunity), which is a very demanding protein-caloric process, compared with a specific immune response.[54] Therefore, any illness, but in particular chronic, active processes will result in growth retardation or weight loss.

Ensuring animals are healthy before departure using a clinical examination is another key consideration. Specifically, animals with umbilical infections, dehydration, diarrhea, or respiratory disease should not be allowed to get transported. Following a specific clinical examination will not only allow for the detection of diseased animals in a timely manner to improve cure rates at the dairy farm, but it will also avoid the introduction of infections and poor performing animals into the veal and dairy-beef herd.

Assuring sufficient uptake of colostral antibodies is crucial. The general recommendation is, as in female dairy calves, the higher the level of IgG the better. In **Table 1**, suggestions for potential cut-offs for calf purchasing and preconditioning programs are given based on the recent consensus and available veal studies discussed above.

Table 1
Potential factors for a preconditioning program for male dairy calves destined for the veal and dairy beef industry

Factor[a]	Recommendation
Body weight	>50 kg (>110 lbs) for a Holstein calf, independent from age
Clinical examination	No abnormal clinical signs: fever, cough (including induced cough (reflex), tachypnea/dyspnea, nasal or ocular discharge, diarrhea, lameness, or dehydration
Colostrum uptake	In the first week of life: >10 g/L IgG >51 g/L serum protein Between 2 and 4 weeks old: >7.5 g/L IgG
Vaccination	Born from dams vaccinated for the most prevalent respiratory and intestinal pathogens Vaccinated on the farm of origin with transport only after the onset of immunity
Transport	Limited to 8 h without rest Directly to the farm of destination without passage at an auction market or sorting center
Mycoplasma bovis and bovine viral diarrhea virus	Do not commingling calves from positive herds with calves from negative herds in the same veal/dairy beef facility

[a] Factors are ranked according to prioritization based on expected relative impact and achievability in the short term.

Testing for FPTI is best done between days 2 and 9, and in every calf on the dairy farm of origin. Alternatively, in the transition process and to reduce costs, the veal and dairy beef sector can systematically test a subset of calves on arrival, providing regular feedback to the farms of origin. In the EU, calves arrive at an older age necessitating the use of more expensive Ig(G) determination over serum protein.[45] It is outside the scope to review all factors contributing to a successful transfer of passive immunity, which is available elsewhere.[43]

Vaccinating calves before departure from the dairy farm of origin allows for calves to have specific immunity for the most important pathogens before they arrive at the veal/dairy beef facility. Specifically, calves with antibodies for bovine respiratory syncytial virus or bovine coronavirus have lower BRD risk in the first weeks after arrival at the veal operation.[45] Generally, there are 2 options to successfully vaccinate calves before departure to the veal industry[1]: Vaccination of the dams combined with successful colostrum management or[2] vaccinating the calves either intranasally or intramuscularly if sufficient time on the farm of origin is available. For several respiratory pathogens, it has been shown in settings other than the veal industry, that vaccination of the dam increases antibody levels in the calves if colostrum delivery was sufficient, reducing the BRD risk.[55] With respect to vaccinating calves before leaving the source dairy farm, few studies have been conducted. Vertenten and others[56] found that calves provided with an inactivated vaccine for RSV, PI-3, and *Mannheimia haemolytica* and another vaccine for rotavirus, coronavirus, and enterotoxic *Escherichia coli*, had a 6% lower BRD risk in the first days after arrival and an 8% lower mortality risk after they arrived at veal facilities. With the available intranasal vaccines in the EU (RSV and PI-3), vaccination is possible between 7 and 10 days of age, meaning that the onset of immunity is often just reached around departure to the veal farm. Given that a strong seasonal effect is present for BRSV and PI-3 with an epidemic occurring each year between November and April, peaking in January–February, for economic reasons vaccination could be planned in this period.[57] Whether vaccination against opportunistic *Pasteurellaceae* is beneficial for the veal/dairy beef industry is currently unknown. An important limitation to any vaccine program is that no effective vaccine for the dominant pathogen, *M. bovis*, is currently available. The development of a vaccine for *M. bovis* would certainly be a game changer if protective immunity could be reached before arrival at the veal facility.

In the absence of effective vaccination programs for crucial pathogens, an alternative preventive strategy is determining the infectious status of the herds of origin, in particular for *M. bovis* and bovine viral diarrhea virus.[27] The goal of this approach would be to organize calf supply in such a way that calves from *M. bovis* and BVDv-free herds go to the same veal facility and are no longer commingled with calves from positive dairy farms. Despite that the potential benefit, practical organization, and associated costs may be substantial. In the EU, several countries already have a national eradication program for BVDv, but *M. bovis* is currently thriving in the dairy industry with a prevalence of around 20% to 30% of the farms.[28] A recent study showed that rather than evidence for persistence of *M. bovis* in the veal industry, new strains are systematically imported from the dairy industry in each veal production round.[58]

Limiting the number of herds of origin could also be a strategy to reduce disease pressure. However, it would be difficult to achieve in the veal/dairy beef industry due to the size of the veal farms relative to the dairy farms. In small scale veal farming in Switzerland, herds that did not purchase had lower antimicrobial use and mortality.[59] In addition, in a Canadian study, calves derived from an auction facility had a higher risk of mortality than calves from local dairy farms highlighting the benefit of direct transportation.[34] Likely more evidence on the effects of directly transporting to the veal herd or avoiding substantial commingling and additional stress at sorting centers or auction markets will be needed to change this inherent element of the veal and dairy beef industry.

Transport is a significant contributor to increasing disease susceptibility and is very sensitive to criticism by the public, especially in young animals.[60] Besides a single study evidencing that calves with higher body weight cope better with short transport, studies on the effect of transport in neonatal calves are lacking.[41] Several aspects to improve transport need to be evaluated including time in transport, bedding and space provision, and access to feeders and drinkers. From studies in beef cattle, it should be highlighted that shorter transport times and resting periods are beneficial for stress and disease risk.[51] Studies on transport, the associated stress, and disease risk and effects of preconditioning are an important research gap to make the veal and dairy beef industry more sustainable in the future.

Finally, even if ensuring that only calves of higher quality (ie, body weight at arrival >50 kg (>110 lbs), serum IgG level greater than 10 g/L, and no clinical abnormalities) looks straightforward, in many countries it will be difficult. Producers should be encouraged to establish relationships locally with dairy producers to minimize the length of time in transit, but also consider providing monetary incentives to those that provide high-quality calves.[61] Benchmarking mortality, morbidity, and FTPI levels for each source dairy farm of origin could also serve as a means of encouraging changes to calf management practices and ultimately improve the quality of calves being received.[62]

Managing Newly Arrived Calves at Veal or Dairy-Beef Facilities

Clearly, how calves are managed after calves arrive at the veal or dairy beef facility can have a substantial influence on mortality and morbidity.[34] In addition, it is unlikely that the proposed changes highlighted above will occur rapidly due to the multiple stakeholders that are involved in the decision-making process. Therefore, management practices within the current system need to be put into place to ensure mortality and morbidity are minimized. In addition, even if every measure is in place to ensure the entry of excellent quality calves, it is still likely that "high-risk calves" will enter the facility. Hence, efforts should be made to identify high-risk calves which could include a 30-sec examination of the calf to determine if the calf is dehydrated or has diarrhea, a depressed attitude, depressed paralumbar fossa, or an umbilical infection. When calves are identified with dehydration or diarrhea, it may be prudent to provide an oral electrolyte to restore fluid and electrolyte balance, whereas calves with an umbilical infection should be treated with an injectable antimicrobial. Although this approach has not been well validated, it could be used to reduce the risk of disease and mortality in high-risk calves. Beyond these clinical parameters, calves with a body weight at arrival less than 50 kg (<110 lbs) could also be identified as high-risk; however, it is unclear the nutritional strategies or management practices that should be put in place to minimize disease risk. In a recent study a cluster analysis differentiated high from low-risk calves based on arrival parameters.[48] Low-risk calves had an above-average body weight and immunoglobulin concentration and a below-average concentration of acute phase proteins and cortisol. Reversely, high-risk calves had low bodyweight, low immunoglobulin levels, mounted an acute phase response, and had higher cortisol.[48] Whether clustering on many different blood parameters eventually is economically justifiable, remains to be determined.

A management practice that has traditionally been implemented to minimize disease risk is the use of antimicrobials on arrival to the calf-raising facility. Although it has been commonly used, with 56% of calf ranches and 14% of dairy farms in the United States using medicated milk replacer,[63,64] in the literature the efficacy of this practice is variable. Of the studies that have found positive effects, most of the response to oral antimicrobials lead to minor reductions in fecal consistency score and number of days with diarrhea (17 d with oral antimicrobials compared with 19 days without)[65–67] or days with antimicrobial treatment (0.3 d with oral antimicrobials compared with 1.1 day without).[68] One study identified that calves receiving antimicrobials in milk replacer had lower mortality and morbidity compared with calves that did not receive antimicrobials.[69] It is important to note, however, that most of these studies fed low levels of milk[65,66,69] and some of the diarrhea could have been related to nutrition.[66] In addition, in some of these studies, the oral antimicrobials had similar effects to the provision of a prebiotic.[65,66] Of note other studies that have fed antimicrobials have either found no effect[68] or even an increased risk of diarrhea.[70–72] Given the mixed results, the provision of antimicrobials to calves on arrival requires reconsideration and alternatives should be sought especially as in different EU countries, starting with the Netherlands and Belgium, systematic pro-/metaphylactic antimicrobial use on arrival is forbidden.

In many veal and dairy beef facilities to accustom calves to new housing and nutrition, feeding is restricted in the first days. Besides empiric experience, there are no studies available evaluating the benefits of this strategy. Given that a substantial number of calves arrive malnourished, the provision of a higher volume of milk fed to calves should be considered. Several studies have found that offering ≥ 20% of their BW per day (by volume) in milk leads to improved immune function,[73,74] faster recovery from diarrhea,[75] reduced cases of diarrhea,[76] and reduced disease treatment in the pre-weaning period[77] compared with restricted (≤10% BW) planes of nutrition. Improved preweaning growth rates and feed efficiency will also result from high milk feeding programs compared with restricted levels of milk.[78–80] In addition, calves will display less signs of behavioral indicators of hunger and reduce the number of vocalizations when provided a higher nutritional plane.[81] Hence, producers raising veal or dairy-beef calves should strive to eliminate the use of restricted planes of nutrition to improve calf health, welfare, and growth.

Beyond improving the nutritional plane, the addition of additives to milk may also have value. A narrative review highlighted that the strategic use of probiotics and prebiotics could lead to improved health, mostly through reduced diarrhea risk in male and female dairy calves.[82] This was found to be particularly true when disease challenge was highly similar to what is seen at veal and dairy-beef farms. Furthermore, most advantages were seen when yeast or bacterial-based probiotics were supplemented. Other additives that could be used include spray-dried plasma protein which has been shown to reduce diarrhea and calf mortality likely due to the high concentration of immunoglobulins, growth factors, and other functional proteins that could improve intestinal health.[83–86] Prolonged supplementation of colostrum replacer or pasteurized colostrum in milk has also been shown to be an effective strategy to improve calf health. Specifically, providing colostrum replacer or pasteurized colostrum for 14 days after first colostrum feeding has been shown to improve health scores, reduce the number of days with diarrhea, respiratory disease, and antimicrobial treatments, and lead to improved growth.[87–89] With respect to saturated and unsaturated fatty acid esters supplemented from arrival at a veal facility, there was no improvement in health and production found.[90,91]

Due to the rise of certain resistant bacteria, such as *Salmonella* Dublin,[92] the implementation of biosecurity practices is especially critical to prevent the entry of pathogens, control outbreaks, and reduce the cyclicity of pathogens within a facility. Despite its importance, the application of biosecurity measures is low within the veal industry.[93] The use of an all-in all-out system has been highlighted as one biosecurity practice that can lead to lower disease levels whereby all animals are brought into a facility within a short period of time, all animals are sent out at the same time, and cleaning and disinfecting occurs between groups. Specifically, having a clean and disinfected environment for calf housing has been shown to reduce the presence of several pathogens such as *Salmonella*.[94] Implementation of herd-specific clothing and footwear for veterinarians and other professional advisors is likely also critical to prevent the spread to the farm, but also to other clients they serve. Staff can serve as a vector for disease spread so ensuring that coveralls are cleaned frequently and working from the youngest to oldest animals on the farm can help to limit disease spread.

The most accessible route of vaccination in the veal/dairy beef industry is vaccination on or shortly after arrival. However, at that time animals are severely stressed, and the pathogens are already spreading, theoretically meaning that the infection will be earlier than the onset of immunity. In a single observational study from Switzerland, a reduced mortality was shown in vaccinating veal herds.[59] Few randomized clinical trials are available. An Italian study on intranasal vaccination against RSV and PI-3 in 2136 veal calves showed a reduction in lung lesion score, but no effects on growth and mortality.[95] In a calf rearing facility in Finland, intranasally vaccinated calves had a greater average daily gain, but no reduced morbidity.[96] In addition, due to the high levels of maternally derived antibodies when calves arrive at veal and dairy-beef facilities in North America, parenteral vaccines at arrival are discouraged and veal/dairy beef trials are lacking to prove otherwise.[97] Hence, more studies on vaccination in the function of the veal/dairy beef industry are needed. Incorporating thoracic ultrasonography and an etiologic diagnosis of respiratory disease would improve the quality of randomized controlled trials on this topic, which are urgently needed.

With respect to housing, a recent review by Ollivett[98] highlighted that there are mixed results with respect to housing strategies. However, small group sizes or individual housing may lessen the impact of respiratory disease compared with groups that are larger than 5 to 10 calves. Others have also highlighted the importance of stocking density, air pollutants, and ventilation which play a critical role in preventing respiratory disease but fall outside the scope of the present article.[99–101]

SUMMARY

Veal, dairy beef, and dairy industries need to economically work together, meaning reasonable prices for good quality calves with reduced disease risk. Only this will result in a sustainable reduction of antimicrobial use and increase production and welfare, to the benefit of all industries and society. Rather than legal criteria on transport age, a practical regulatory framework may be a 50 kg (110 lbs) body weight for transport criterion from the dairy farm of origin as its association with disease is evidenced and the parameter is easy to control in contrast to age determination. Vaccination and transport studies are absolute research priorities to give the present production system a chance for a license to produce in the future.

DISCLOSURE

The authors have nothing to disclose.

REFERENCES

1. Creutzinger K, Pempek J, Habing G, et al. Perspectives on the management of surplus dairy calves in the United States and Canada. Front Vet Sci 2021;8: 661453.
2. Canadian Dairy Information Centre. Number of farms, dairy cows, and dairy heifers. 2021. Available at: https://www.dairyinfo.gc.ca/eng/dairy-statistics-and-market-information/farm-statistics/farms-dairy-cows-and-dairy-heifers/?id=1502467423238. Assessed April 15, 2021.
3. United States Department of Agriculture. National agricultural statistics service. Milk cows: inventory by year, US 2021. Available at: https://www.nass.usda.gov/Charts_and_Maps/Milk_Production_and_Milk_Cows/milkcows.php. Assessed April 15, 2021.
4. ADHB. UK and EU cow numbers. 2021. Available at: https://ahdb.org.uk/dairy/uk-and-eu-cow-numbers.
5. De Vries A, Overton M, Fetrow J, et al. Exploring the impact of sexed semen on the structure of the dairy industry. J Dairy Sci 2008;91:847–56.
6. Pardon B, Catry B, Boone R, et al. Characteristics and challenges of the modern Belgian veal industry. Vlaams Diergeneeskd Tijdschr 2014;83:155–63.
7. Eurostat. Agricultural production - livestock and meat. 2020. Available at: https://ec.europa.eu/eurostat/statistics-explained/index.php?title=Agricultural_production_-_livestock_and_meat&oldid=470510#Veal_and_beef. Assessed April 15, 2021.

8. Statistics Canada. Cattle and calves, farm and meat production. 2021. Available at: https://www150.statcan.gc.ca/t1/tbl1/en/tv.action?pid=3210012501. Assessed April 15, 2021.
9. Berry D. Invited review: Beef-on-dairy - The generation of crossbred beef x dairy cattle. J Dairy Sci 2021;104:3789–819.
10. Ettema J, Thomasen J, Hjortø L, et al. Economic opportunities for using sexed semen and semen of beef bulls in dairy herds. J Dairy Sci 2017;100:4161–71.
11. Les Producteurs de bovins du Québec. Price-Info - Cull cattle and dairy calves. 2021. Available at: http://bovin.qc.ca/en/price-info/cull-cattle-and-bob-calves/weekly/. Assessed April 15, 2021.
12. de Vries M, van Middelaar C, de Boer I. Comparing environmental impacts of beef production systems: A review of life cycle assessments. Livest Sci 2015;178:279–88.
13. Bolton S, von Keyserlingk M. The dispensable surplus dairy calf: is this issue a "wicked problem" and where do we go from here? Front Vet Sci 2021;8:660934.
14. Rutherford NH, Lively FO, Arnott G. A review of beef production systems for the sustainable use of surplus male dairy-origin calves within the UK. Front Vet Sci 2021;8:635497.
15. Wilson LL, Egan CL, Henning WR, et al. Effects of live animal performance and hemoglobin level on special-fed veal carcass characteristics. Meat Sci 1995;41:89–96.
16. Leruste H, Brscic M, Cozzi G, et al. Prevalence and potential influencing factors of non-nutritive oral behaviors of veal calves on commercial farms. J Dairy Sci 2014;97:7021–30.
17. Pardon B, Catry B, Dewulf J, et al. Prospective study on quantitative and qualitative antimicrobial and anti-inflammatory drug use in white veal calves. J Antimicrob Chemother 2012;67:1027–38.
18. Bokma J, Boone R, Deprez P, et al. Risk factors for antimicrobial use in veal calves and the association with mortality. J Dairy Sci 2019;102:607–18.
19. BelVet-Sac. Belgian Veterinary Surveillance of Antimicrobial Consumption National Consumption Report. 2020. Available at: https://belvetsac.ugent.be/BelvetSac_report_2019.pdf.
20. Catry B, Haesebrouck F, Vliegher SD, et al. Variability in acquired resistance of Pasteurella and Mannheimia isolates from the nasopharynx of calves, with particular reference to different herd types. Microb Drug Resist 2005;11:387–94.
21. Catry B, Dewulf J, Maes D, et al. Effect of antimicrobial consumption and production type on antibacterial resistance in the bovine respiratory and digestive tract. PLoS One 2016;11:e0146488.
22. Bos ME, Graveland H, Portengen L, et al. Livestock-associated MRSA prevalence in veal calf production is associated with farm hygiene, use of antimicrobials, and age of the calves. Prev Vet Med 2012;105:155–9.
23. Hordijk J, Wagenaar JA, Kant A, et al. Cross-sectional study on prevalence and molecular characteristics of plasmid mediated ESBL/AmpC-producing Escherichia coli isolated from veal calves at slaughter. PLoS One 2013;8:e65681.
24. Landers T, Cohen B, Wittum T, et al. A review of antibiotic use in food animals: Perspective, policy, and potential. Public Health Rep 2012;127:4–22.
25. Pardon B, Hostens M, Duchateau L, et al. Impact of respiratory disease, diarrhea, otitis and arthritis on mortality and carcass traits in white veal calves. BMC Vet Res 2013;9:79.
26. Arcangioli MA, Duet A, Meyer G, et al. The role of Mycoplasma bovis in bovine respiratory disease outbreaks in veal calf feedlots. Vet J 2018;177:89–93.

27. Pardon B, De Bleecker K, Dewulf J, et al. Prevalence of respiratory pathogens in diseased, non-vaccinated, routinely medicated veal calves. Vet Rec 2011; 169:278.

28. Gille L, Callens J, Supre K, et al. Use of a breeding bull and absence of a calving pen as risk factors for the presence of Mycoplasma bovis in dairy herds. J Dairy Sci 2018;101:8284–90.

29. Hulbert L, Moisà S. Stress, immunity, and the management of calves. J Dairy Sci 2016;99:3199–216.

30. Bähler C, Steiner A, Luginbühl A, et al. Risk factors for death and unwanted early slaughter in Swiss veal calves kept at a specific animal welfare standard. Res Vet Sci 2012;92:162–8.

31. Marquou S, Blouin L, Djakite H, et al. Health parameters and their association with price in young calves sold at auction for veal operations in Québec, Canada. J Dairy Sci 2019;102:6454–65.

32. Pempek J, Trearchis D, Masterson M, et al. Veal calf health on the day of arrival at growers in Ohio. J Anim Sci 2017;95:3863–72.

33. Scott K, Kelton D, Duffield T, et al. Risk factors identified on arrival associated with morbidity and mortality at a grain-fed veal facility: A prospective, single-cohort study. J Dairy Sci 2019;102:9224–35.

34. Renaud D, Duffield T, LeBlanc S, et al. Risk factors associated with mortality at a milk-fed veal calf facility: A prospective cohort study. J Dairy Sci 2018;101:2659–68.

35. Wilson D, Stojkov J, Renaud D, et al. Short communication: Condition of male dairy calves at auction markets. J Dairy Sci 2020;103:8530–4.

36. Wilson D, Stojkov J, Renaud D, et al. Risk factors for poor health outcomes for male dairy calves undergoing transportation in western Canada. Can Vet J 2020;61:1265–72.

37. Renaud D, Overton M, Dhuyvetter K, et al. Effect of health status evaluated at arrival on growth in milk-fed veal calves: A prospective single cohort study. J Dairy Sci 2018;101:10383–90.

38. Marcato F, van den Brand H, Kemp B, et al. Evaluating potential biomarkers of health and performance in veal calves. Front Vet Sci 2018;5:133.

39. Brscic M, Leruste H, Heutinck L, et al. Prevalence of respiratory disorders in veal calves and potential risk factors. J Dairy Sci 2012;95:2753–64.

40. Goetz H, Kelton D, Costa J, et al. Identification of biomarkers measured upon arrival associated with morbidity, mortality, and average daily gain in grain-fed veal calves. J Dairy Sci 2021;104:874–85.

41. Masmeijer C, Devriendt B, Rogge T, et al. Randomized field trial on the effects of body weight and short transport on stress and immune variables in 2-to 4-week-old dairy calves. J Vet Intern Med 2019;33:1514–29.

42. Renaud D, Duffield T, LeBlanc S, et al. Clinical and metabolic indicators associated with early mortality at a milk-fed veal facility: A prospective case-control study. J Dairy Sci 2018;101:2669–78.

43. Godden S, Lombard J, Woolums A. Colostrum management for dairy calves. Vet Clin North Am Food Anim Pract 2019;35:535–56.

44. Wilson L, Smith J, Smith D, et al. Characteristics of veal calves upon arrival, at 28 and 84 days, and at end of the production cycle. J Dairy Sci 2000;83:843–54.

45. Pardon B, Alliët J, Boone R, et al. Prediction of respiratory disease and diarrhea in veal calves based on immunoglobulin levels and serostatus for respiratory pathogens measured at arrival. Prev Vet Med 2015;120:169–76.

46. Lombard J, Urie N, Garry F, et al. Consensus recommendations on calf- and herd-level passive immunity in dairy calves in the United States. J Dairy Sci 2020;103:7611–24.

47. Wilm J, Costa J, Neave H, et al. Technical note: Serum total protein and immunoglobulin G concentrations in neonatal dairy calves over the first 10 days of age. J Dairy Sci 2018;101:6430–6.

48. Masmeijer C, Deprez P, van Leenen K, et al. Arrival cortisol measurement in veal calves and its association with body weight, protein fractions, animal health and performance. Prev Vet Med 2021;187:105251.

49. Earley B, Buckham Sporer K, Gupta S. Invited review: Relationship between cattle transport, immunity and respiratory disease. Animal 2017;11:486–92.

50. Holland BP, Burciaga-Robles LO, VanOverbeke DL, et al. Effect of bovine respiratory disease during preconditioning on subsequent feedlot performance, carcass characteristics, and beef attributes. J Anim Sci 2010;88:2486–99.

51. Melendez DM, Marti S, Haley DB, et al. Effects of conditioning, source, and rest on indicators of stress in beef cattle transported by road. PLoS One 2021;16: e0244854.

52. Alharthi AS, Coleman DN, Alhidary IA, et al. Maternal body condition during late-pregnancy is associated with in utero development and neonatal growth of Holstein calves. J Anim Sci Biotechnol 2021;12:44.

53. Hall JA, Bobe G, Vorachek WR, et al. Effect of supranutritional maternal and colostral selenium supplementation on passive absorption of immunoglobulin G in selenium-replete dairy calves. J Dairy Sci 2014;97:4379–91.

54. Otalora-Ardila A, Herrera ML, Flores-Martinez JJ, et al. Metabolic Cost of the Activation of Immune Response in the Fish-Eating Myotis (Myotis vivesi): The Effects of Inflammation and the Acute Phase Response. PLoS One 2016;11: e0164938.

55. Makoschey B, Ramage C, Reddick D, et al. Colostrum from cattle immunized with a vaccine based on iron regulated proteins of Mannheimia haemolytica confers partial protection. Vaccine 2012;30:969–73.

56. Vertenten, G., Chanteperdrix, M., Mounaix, B., Guiadeur, M., Martineau, C., Assié, S., Masselin, S., Le Nouvel, C., Leboeuf, F., Jozan, T. Health and production benefits in veal calves born from NCD and BRD vaccinated cows. Abstracts of the European Buiatrics Congres. 2020. September 11th-13th, s' Hertogenbosch, The Netherlands.

57. Pardon B, Callens J, Maris J, et al. Pathogen-specific risk factors in acute outbreaks of respiratory disease in calves. J Dairy Sci 2020;103:2556–66.

58. Bokma J, Vereecke N, De Bleecker K, et al. Phylogenomic analysis of Mycoplasma bovis from Belgian veal, dairy and beef herds. Vet Res 2020;51:121.

59. Lava M, Schüpbach-Regula G, Steiner A, et al. Antimicrobial drug use and risk factors associated with treatment incidence and mortality in Swiss veal calves reared under improved welfare conditions. Prev Vet Med 2016;126:121–30.

60. Buddle EA, Bray HJ, Ankeny RA. "I feel sorry for them": australian meat consumers' perceptions about sheep and beef cattle transportation. Animals 2018;8:171.

61. Ventura B, Weary D, Giovanetti A, et al. Veterinary perspectives on cattle welfare challenges and solutions. Livest Sci 2016;193:95–102.

62. Sumner C, von Keyserlingk M, Weary D. How benchmarking motivates farmers to improve dairy calf management. J Dairy Sci 2018;101:3323–33.

63. Walker W, Epperson W, Wittum T, et al. Characteristics of dairy calf ranches: Morbidity, mortality, antibiotic use practices, and biosecurity and biocontainment practices. J Dairy Sci 2012;95:2204–14.

64. Urie N, Lombard J, Shivley C, et al. Preweaned heifer management on US dairy operations: Part I. Descriptive characteristics of preweaned heifer raising practices. J Dairy Sci 2018;101:9168–84.

65. Quigley J, Drewry J, Murray L, et al. Body weight gain, feed efficiency, and fecal scores of dairy calves in response to galactosyl-lactose or antibiotics in milk replacers. J Dairy Sci 1997;80:1751–4.

66. Heinrichs A, Jones C, Heinrichs B. Effects of mannan oligosaccharide or antibiotics in neonatal diets on health and growth of dairy calves. J Dairy Sci 2003;86:4064–9.

67. Buss L, Yohe T, Cangiano L, et al. The effect of neomycin inclusion in milk replacer on the health, growth, and performance of male Holstein calves preweaning. J Dairy Sci 2021;104(7):8188–201.

68. Dennis T, Suarez-Mena F, Hu W, et al. Effects of milk replacer feeding rate and long-term antibiotic inclusion in milk replacer on performance and nutrient digestibility of Holstein dairy calves up to 4 months of age. J Dairy Sci 2019;102:2094–102.

69. Berge A, Lindeque P, Moore D, et al. A clinical trial evaluating prophylactic and therapeutic antibiotic use on health and performance of preweaned calves. J Dairy Sci 2005;88:2166–77.

70. Berge A, Moore D, Besser T, et al. Targeting therapy to minimize antimicrobial use in preweaned calves: Effects on health, growth, and treatment costs. J Dairy Sci 2009;92:4707–14.

71. Mero K, Rollin R, Phillips R. Malabsorption due to selected oral antibiotics. Vet Clin North Am Food Anim Pract 1985;1:581–8.

72. Shull J, Frederick H. Adverse effect of oral antibacterial prophylaxis and therapy on incidence of neonatal calf diarrhea. Vet Med Small Anim Clin 1978;73:924–30.

73. Ballou M. Immune responses of Holstein and Jersey calves during the preweaning and immediate postweaned periods when fed varying planes of milk replacer. J Dairy Sci 2012;95:7319–30.

74. Ballou M, Hanson D, Cobb C, et al. Plane of nutrition influences the performance, innate leukocyte response, and resistance to an oral *Salmonella enterica* serotype Typhimurium challenge in Jersey calves. J Dairy Sci 2015;98:1972–82.

75. Ollivett T, Nydam D, Linden T, et al. Effect of nutritional plane on health and performance in dairy calves after experimental infection with *Cryptosporidium parvum*. J Am Vet Med Assoc 2012;241:1514–20.

76. Khan M, Lee H, Lee W, et al. Pre- and postweaning performance of Holstein female calves fed milk through step-down and conventional methods. J Dairy Sci 2007;90:876–85.

77. Todd C, Millman S, Leslie K, et al. Effects of milk replacer acidification and free-access feeding on early life feeding, oral, and lying behaviour of dairy calves. J Dairy Sci 2018;101:8236–47.

78. Appleby M, Weary D, Chua B. Performance and feeding behaviour of calves on ad libitum milk from artificial teats. Appl Anim Behav Sci 2001;74:191–201.

79. Rosenberger K, Costa J, Neave H, et al. The effect of milk allowance on behaviour and weight gains in dairy calves. J Dairy Sci 2017;100:504–12.

80. Bartlett S, Mckeith F, Vandeharr M, et al. Growth and body composition of dairy calves fed milk replacers. J Anim Sci 2006;84:1454.
81. Thomas T, Weary D, Appleby M. Newborn and 5-week-old calves vocalize in response to milk deprivation. Appl Anim Behav Sci 2001;74:165–73.
82. Cangiano L, Yohe T, Steele M, et al. Invited Review: Strategic use of microbial-based probiotics and prebiotics in dairy calf rearing. Appl Anim Sci 2020;36: 630–51.
83. Quigley J, Drew M. Effects of oral antibiotics or bovine plasma on survival, health and growth in dairy calves challenged with *Escherichia coli*. Food Agric Immunol 2000;12:311–8.
84. Quigley J, Wolfe T. Effects of spray-dried animal plasma in calf milk replacer on health and growth of dairy calves. J Dairy Sci 2003;86:586–92.
85. Wood D, Blome R, Keunen A, et al. Short communication: Effects of porcine plasma or combined sodium butyrate and *Bacillus subtilis* on growth and health of grain-fed veal calves. J Dairy Sci 2019;102:7183–8.
86. Thornsberry R, Wood D, Kertz A, et al. Alternative ingredients in calf milk replacer - A review for bovine practitioners. Bov Pract 2016;50:65–88.
87. Berge A, Besser T, Moore D, et al. Evaluation of the effects of oral colostrum supplementation during the first fourteen days on the health and performance of preweaned calves. J Dairy Sci 2009;92:286–95.
88. Chamorro M, Cernicchiaro N, Haines D. Evaluation of the effects of colostrum replacer supplementation of the milk replacer ration on the occurrence of disease, antibiotic therapy, and performance of pre-weaned dairy calves. J Dairy Sci 2016;100:1378–87.
89. Kargar S, Roshan M, Ghoreishi S, et al. Extended colostrum feeding for 2 weeks improves growth performance and reduces the susceptibility to diarrhea and pneumonia in neonatal Holstein dairy calves. J Dairy Sci 2020;103:8130–42.
90. Masmeijer C, Rogge T, van Leenen K, et al. Effects of glycerol-esters of saturated short- and medium chain fatty acids on immune, health and growth variables in veal calves. Prev Vet Med 2020;178:104983.
91. Masmeijer C, van Leenen K, De Cremer L, et al. Effects of omega-3 fatty acids on immune, health and growth variables in veal calves. Prev Vet Med 2020;179: 104979.
92. Holschbach C, Peek S. *Salmonella* in dairy cattle. Vet Clin North Am Food Anim Pract 2018;34:133–54.
93. Damiaans B, Renault V, Sarrazin S, et al. Biosecurity practices in Belgian veal calf farming: Level of implementation, attitudes, strengths, weaknesses and constraints. Prev Vet Med 2019;172:104768.
94. Fossler C, Wells S, Kaneene J, et al. Herd-level factors associated with isolation of Salmonella in a multi-state study of conventional and organic dairy farms: I. Salmonella shedding in cows. Prev Vet Med 2005;70:257–77.
95. Cavirani S, Taddei S, Cabassi C, et al. Field study on an intranasal vaccination protocol in veal calf farms. Large Anim Rev 2016;22:51–6.
96. Sandelin A, Härtel H, Seppä-Lassila L, et al. Field trial to evaluate the effect of an intranasal respiratory vaccine protocol on bovine respiratory incidence and growth in a commercial rearing unit. BMC Vet Res 2020;16:73.
97. Woolums A, Berghaus R, Berghaus L, et al. Effect of calf age and administration route of initial multivalent modified-live virus vaccine on humoral and cell-mediated immune responses following subsequent administration of a booster vaccination at weaning in beef calves. Am J Vet Res 2013;74:343–54.

98. Ollivett T. How does housing influence bovine respiratory disease in dairy and veal calves? Vet Clin North Am Food Anim Pract 2020;36:385–98.

99. van Leenen K, Jouret J, Demeyer P, et al. Associations of barn air quality parameters with ultrasonographic lung lesions, airway inflammation and infection in group-housed calves. Prev Vet Med 2020a;181:105056.

100. van Leenen K, Jouret J, Demeyer P, et al. Particulate matter and airborne endotoxin concentration in calf barns and their association with lung consolidation, inflammation, and infection. J Dairy Sci 2021;104:5932–47.

101. Nordlund K, Halbach C. Calf barn design to optimize health and ease of management. Vet Clin North Am Food Anim Pract 2019;35:29–45.

Bovine Respiratory Disease Considerations in Young Dairy Calves

Daniel B. Cummings, DVM[a,*],
Nathan F. Meyer, MS, MBA, PhD, DVM[a,b,1],
Douglas L. Step, DVM, DACVIM[a,2]

KEYWORDS

- Bovine respiratory disease complex • Risk factors • Metaphylaxis • Treatment

KEY POINTS

- Bovine respiratory disease is the second leading cause of morbidity in preweaned dairy calves and leading cause of morbidity in weaned dairy calves.
- Assessing and managing risks associated with BRD in commercial dairy calves is an important aspect of controlling morbidity and mortality.
- Veterinarians must work with caretakers to ensure timely and accurate diagnosis of respiratory disease by implementing advanced screening and diagnostic tools.
- Treatment and control of BRD has focused on antimicrobial therapy, which is efficacious when applied early in disease progression and in the correct population.

INTRODUCTION

Bovine respiratory disease (BRD) is a multifactorial disease complex resulting in the development of bronchopneumonia or pleuropneumonia. Respiratory disease impacts multiple segments of the beef and dairy industries. This complex disease affects dairy and dairy-beef cross calves and is commonly referred to as dairy calf pneumonia or enzootic calf pneumonia. Results from the 2011 US National Animal Health Monitoring Survey (NAHMS) revealed that pneumonia is a major cause of morbidity affecting preweaned (18.1%) and weaned (11.2%) dairy replacement heifers.[1]

Negative impacts associated with BRD in commercial dairy raising operations may cause short-term and long-term losses. Costs of respiratory disease include labor, reduced performance (short-term and long-term), animal replacement costs, and

[a] Boehringer Ingelheim Animal Health USA Inc., 3239 Satellite Blvd., Duluth, GA, 30096;
[b] Affiliate Faculty, Department of Clinical Sciences, Colorado State University, 1601 Campus Delivery, Fort Collins, CO, 80523
[1] Present address: 3239 Satellite Blvd., Duluth GA, 30096
[2] Present address: 3239 Satellite Blvd., Duluth GA, 30096
* Corresponding author. PO Box 1599, Hopkinsville, KY 42240.
E-mail address: dbc0006@gmail.com

Vet Clin Food Anim 38 (2022) 93–105
https://doi.org/10.1016/j.cvfa.2021.11.007
0749-0720/22/© 2021 Elsevier Inc. All rights reserved.
vetfood.theclinics.com

veterinary fees. Dairy or dairy-beef cross cattle affected with BRD in the finishing phase of production may have decreased marbling, decreased average daily gain (ADG), decreased quality grade, and increased mortality similar to that observed in native beef cattle.[2] Research has demonstrated that calfhood pneumonia affecting dairy heifers may decrease weight gain, age at first service and hence calving, increase culling risk, and lower future milk production.[3] An economic analysis in 2021 estimated the cost of BRD in dairy replacement females occurring in the first 120 days of age to be $252 or $282, depending on future milk production for replacement females.[3]

The impact of BRD for commercial dairy calf raisers may vary depending on a multitude of factors including the accuracy and completeness of disease detection and effectiveness of applied treatments.[3] The goal of this article is to provide the practitioner a practical reference on the BRD complex, current diagnostics and discuss approaches to using antimicrobials to treat and control BRD in young dairy calves.

REVIEW OF BRD COMPLEX

Calf pneumonia involves several host-environment-pathogen interactions. Interactions that suppress or interfere with host defense mechanisms increase the risk of BRD in young calves due to impairment of immunologic and physiologic responses.[4] The host immune system can be affected by concurrent disease, dehydration, genetics, nutritional deficiencies or imbalances, surgical procedures, and chronic stress. Recognized environmental factors contributing to the increased risk of respiratory disease include poor ventilation, inadequate bedding, overcrowding, inclement weather, transportation, and other causes of stress.[4] Chronic stress in cattle results in suppression of the acute-phase response modulated by the transient release of cortisol.[5] This immunosuppressive response may allow respiratory pathogens access to the lower respiratory tract resulting in pneumonia.[6]

VIRAL INFECTION

Primary viral infections can compromise the host resulting in bacterial pneumonia through the following 4 mechanisms: (1) damage to upper respiratory tract mucosa and mucociliary clearance mechanisms; (2) damage to tracheal epithelial cells resulting in bacterial attachment, growth, and colonization; (3) depletion or damage to innate host defense mechanisms in the airways and lungs including macrophages and neutrophils required for phagocytosis of foreign invaders; and (4) suppression of the acquired immune system including both cell-mediated and humoral responses.[7]

Generally, bovine viral diarrhea virus (BVDV), parainfluenza-3 virus, bovine respiratory syncytial virus, and bovine herpesvirus type 1 are considered primary viral respiratory pathogens; it is commonly recommended that respiratory vaccines contain some or all of these antigens.[7] Infection with BVDV is known to contribute to clinical BRD depending on virulence factors, acute/transient or persistent infection, time of exposure, and presence of secondary pathogens.[8] Therefore, BVDV control strategies are warranted to effectively control BRD in this population of calves.

Recently, bovine coronavirus, influenza D virus, and bovine adenovirus have been isolated from clinical cases and included in diagnostic reports.[4,9] The role of these agents as primary respiratory tract infections has not yet been clearly defined.

MYCOPLASMA AND OTHER BACTERIAL INFECTIONS

Mannheimia haemolytica, *Pasteurella multocida*, and *Histophilus somni* are the most common bacterial pathogens associated with BRD.[7] Clinical signs attributable to bacterial bronchopneumonia may include anorexia, depression, nasal discharge, tachypnea, and dyspnea depending on the pathogens present. *M haemolytica* is a gram-negative aerobic bacterium, which causes fibrinopurulent bronchopneumonia. Known virulence factors include endotoxin and the production of an exotoxin called leukotoxin. The leukotoxin from *M haemolytica* causes cytolysis of ruminant lymphocytes, macrophages, platelets, and neutrophils.[4] *P multocida* and *H somni* are also gram-negative aerobic bacteria that can be found in the nasopharynx of healthy cattle, similar to *M haemolytica*. However, identification of these pathogens in the nasal passage or nasopharynx does not necessarily result in disease. Moreover, *H somni* can result in septicemia and spread to various organs including the endometrium, joints, heart, and lungs resulting in endometritis, polyarthritis, myocarditis, and pneumonia, respectively. Finally, *Bibersteinia trehalosi* and *Trueperella pyogenes* have occasionally been isolated from pneumonic lungs, especially in chronic cases. The risk of pneumonia caused by *B trehalosi* and *T pyogenes* is not fully understood nor is their significance. A challenging study revealed that lung involvement in 2- to 3-month-old crossbred dairy calves inoculated intratracheally with *B trehalosi* was not increased in inoculated calves as compared with controls. The findings in this study suggest that *B trehalosi* may not be a primary pathogen associated with BRD.[10]

The role of mycoplasmas as causative agents in dairy calf pneumonia is of increasing concern for practitioners. Producers are often challenged with prolonged BRD events refractory to treatment resulting in chronically ill, unthrifty calves. Chronic illness typically associated with mycoplasmas is concerning because of the potential for significant economic losses and negative impact on animal welfare.[11] *Mycoplasma bovis* and *Mycoplasma dispar* are the 2 most significant and commonly reported species in North America.[12] Variation in disease severity is common and includes the following clinical presentations: mastitis, arthritis, tenosynovitis, and "pneumonia-arthritis syndrome."[13] Marked increases in *Mycoplasma* spp. isolation occurred when heifers were grouped, which mirrored increases in isolation of *M haemolytica* in that study.[14] Researchers in Canada isolated *Mycoplasma* spp. and *P multocida* in combination more frequently from transtracheal wash samples in clinician-diagnosed pneumonia cases as compared with controls suggesting synergism between these 2 pathogens.[15] These studies indicate that *Mycoplasma* spp. may be involved in mixed infections.

M bovis is known to have unique characteristics contributing to its virulence. Variable surface proteins or surface lipoproteins expressed by *M bovis* are rapidly activated or deactivated, resulting in extensive genetic and antigenic variation.[11] These variations allow *M bovis* to evade the host defense mechanisms. Variation in surface lipoproteins may also contribute to persistent infections and poor response to vaccination.[16] *M bovis* can initiate proinflammatory cascades mimicking endotoxin-like effects, induce apoptosis of lymphocytes resulting in immunosuppression, and impair both neutrophil and macrophage activity.[4,16] In addition, *Mycoplasma* spp. lack a cell wall. Appreciating these unique characteristics of *M bovis* will assist in prescribing treatment and control options. For example, β-lactams would not be effective as *M bovis* does not have a cell wall.[16] Antimicrobials specifically labeled for the treatment or control of BRD caused by *M bovis* in beef and nonlactating dairy cattle are available. Anecdotal reports from practitioners suggest that successful treatment outcomes may be achieved by early detection and extended duration of therapy.[17]

Exposure to *M bovis* can occur via infected colostrum or milk and through respiratory secretions from infected animals including dams in maternity pens. Managing the proximities of feeding and housing locations is important to successful preventive health programs. Calves with clinical mycoplasmosis shed large quantities of organisms, thus isolating infected calves could reduce transmission. Overcrowding and poor ventilation increase exposure to airborne *M bovis*; therefore, managing stocking density and improving air quality are important control measures. Other control measures include proper sanitization of equipment and facilities, handling sick calves last, all-in, all-out practices, and improving overall health through proper colostrum management and nutrition.[11] Given the lack of controlled experimental data to support vaccination and the tendency for chronic illness attributable to *M bovis*, it is imperative for the practitioner to implement standard principles to prevent and control disease transmission.

EPIDEMIOLOGY AND RISK FACTORS

Practitioners may observe epizootic or enzootic patterns. Herd level median morbidity rates have been reported at 21.6% with a wide range of incidence (0%–57.6%).[18] On-farm BRD case definitions with records ensure early disease detection and monitoring of health events. The agreement in case identification between producer and veterinarian has been investigated and may be poor.[15,19] Practitioners working with commercial dairy raisers should consider respiratory disease screening, training, and diagnostic tools. Early detection and accurate diagnosis of BRD lead to improved outcomes when treatment interventions are applied.

Risk factors associated with BRD in preweaned and weaned dairy calves may be divided into 2 categories: (1) calf-level factors and (2) farm-level factors.[4] **Table 1** lists common risk factors associated with respiratory disease. The contribution fraction of each risk factor to the development of disease may be difficult to quantify and, in many outbreaks, more than one factor may be involved. Certain risk factors such as failure of passive transfer have been identified in multiple studies suggesting these may play a more significant role in the development of BRD.[20] The importance of proper management to minimize risk is too often underscored. Lack of adequate management often results in increased dependence on other management strategies including pharmaceuticals and biologics.

CURRENT DIAGNOSTIC APPROACHES

The approach to diagnosing clinical BRD is traditionally rooted in clinical evaluation/observation of individuals or a group of calves by a caretaker or veterinarian. The observer may identify abnormal behaviors such as depression, lowered head position, head tilt, dyspnea, ocular or nasal discharge, or anorexia. Many of the clinical signs observed with BRD may also be present with other diseases such as septicemia or gastrointestinal disease. Therefore, it is critical for the observers to develop a

Table 1	
Risk factors associated with respiratory disease in commercial dairy calves	
Calf	**Farm**
Failure of passive transfer	Poor ventilation or air quality
Concurrent disease	Housing environment
Navel dipping	Age range at pen level
Nutritional deficiencies	Overcrowding
Vaccination status	Inadequate bedding
Gender	Extreme temperature fluctuations
Surgical procedures	Commingling (All-in, all-out best)

standardized approach for assessing clinical respiratory disease. Furthermore, owing to the discrepancies documented between observers and inaccuracy of detection, it may be beneficial for operations to adopt a more complete diagnostic approach to aid in decision-making processes for treatment. Lastly, confirming a diagnosis of BRD by using proper sampling and diagnostic tests in young dairy calves is of importance provided the increasing pressure on antimicrobial use in food-producing animals.

To aid in the diagnosis, standardized scoring systems for BRD have been developed to assist caretakers and clinicians in their efforts to accurately detect BRD. In feedlots, pen riders commonly use the D.A.R.T system, which stands for depression (D), appetite loss (A), respiratory character change (R), and temperature elevation (T).[21] Advanced scoring systems similar to the D.A.R.T. system can be practically applied in production systems used for raising dairy calves. Two proposed systems evaluated for the screening and diagnosis of BRD in preweaned dairy calves are the California and Wisconsin scoring systems.[22,23] These systems assign a numerical score based on the physical examination and may include temperature, eye score, ear score, cough, head carriage, fecal consistency, navel characteristics, appearance of joints, appetite, depression, nasal discharge, and respirations.[22,24] At least 2 mobile applications have been developed to support caretakers in assigning scores based on clinical signs: The Calf Health Scoring App developed by the University of Wisconsin School of Veterinary Medicine (iTunes App Store) and The UC Davis BRD Scoring App (iTunes App Store). BRD scoring systems present limitations such as screening sensitivity for BRD.[25] These limitations suggest additional screening tests may be necessary to accurately detect clinical BRD and screen for subclinical pneumonia.

Thoracic ultrasonography is an antemortem procedure used to identify pleural effusion, lung consolidation, pleural roughening, or other abnormalities associated with clinical or subclinical bronchopneumonia.[26] Researchers evaluated the accuracy of thoracic ultrasonography to detect subclinical BRD in dairy calves with promising results. A systematic scanning approach to evaluate the right and left lung using specified landmarks demonstrated 94% sensitivity and 100% specificity for the detection of lung lesions.[27] Ollivett and Buczinski describe on-farm thoracic ultrasonography including techniques for detecting BRD in a previous edition.[28] Currently, best practices for screening and diagnosing BRD (clinical or subclinical) in dairy calves use a standardized clinical scoring system concurrently with thoracic ultrasonography.

Microbiologic testing to identify pathogens associated with BRD provides valuable information for the veterinarian to guide prevention and treatment strategies. Practitioners should remember the isolation or detection of specific pathogens must be interpreted carefully. Isolation or detection of pathogens is reliant upon proper sampling and handling techniques. Sampling methods used in dairy calves to detect or isolate respiratory pathogens include transtracheal wash, bronchoalveolar lavage, nasal swab, and guarded nasopharyngeal swab.[29] Pardon and Buczinski provide a thorough review of BRD diagnosis including sampling techniques, diagnostic tests, and interpretation in a previous article.[30]

A necropsy should be considered as part of the diagnostic approach. Valuable information, sample collection, and gross postmortem diagnosis can be obtained. The value of a necropsy is often underappreciated because of economic reasons, time constraints, hesitancy of the clinician, and inconclusive results. Animals may be submitted to veterinary diagnostic laboratories for full necropsy and/or diagnostic tests. In disease outbreaks, it may be warranted to euthanize and submit 2 or more untreated animals with acute clinical signs to obtain meaningful information as opposed to chronic cases.[4]

A cross-sectional study clarifying dairy calf mortalities revealed almost perfect agreement between on-farm necropsy and veterinary diagnostic laboratory results.[31] Gross necropsies performed by veterinarians or personnel with advanced training will provide information to identify certain disease characteristics and limit future losses. A systematic approach when performing gross necropsies is ideal to ensure the investigator identifies all significant abnormalities.[32] Determining the cause of death, concurrent disease, severity, extent, and relative duration of disease allows the practitioner to develop a targeted approach for prevention and treatment of BRD.[33]

TREATMENT AND CONTROL OF BRD

Treatment and control protocols have largely focused on the use of antimicrobials to target the primary bacterial agents involved in BRD. The United States Food and Drug Administration has licensed antimicrobials for the treatment and control of BRD associated with different bacterial pathogens. For the purposes of this article, BRD treatment is defined as therapeutic treatment of an animal following a clinical diagnosis of BRD. Proper identification and diagnosis of BRD is the starting point for treatment. Failure to accurately diagnose subclinical BRD is a primary limitation in the disease management of the young dairy animal.[27] Although numerous antimicrobial options exist for the treatment of BRD, a limited amount of field research data exists when comparing BRD treatment options. One of the key difficulties in conducting BRD treatment trials is a clear case definition and detection. The difficulties associated with conducting BRD treatment trials may explain the relatively few treatment trials compared to control trials in the young dairy calf. BRD control (synonym = metaphylaxis) on a population basis as defined by the American Veterinary Medical Association is as follows:

- Control is the use of antimicrobials to reduce the incidence of infectious disease in a group of animals that already has some individuals with evidence of infectious disease or evidence of infection.[34]

In a practical sense, when an antimicrobial is used for BRD control, animals fall into 1 of the following 3 categories: (1) clinically sick, (2) subclinical, or (3) disease-free but at risk of developing BRD.

Key factors for consideration when using antimicrobials for BRD treatment and control include route of administration, dose, duration of therapy, efficacy, spectrum of activity, protocol adherence, previous experience, and overall economic impact.

BRD Treatment Comparisons

When evaluating therapeutic options for the treatment of BRD, the prospective, masked, randomized clinical trial, in naturally occurring disease is the gold standard.[35] Meta-analyses summarizing BRD treatment and control trials have been published in recent years.[35–38] Meta-analyses are great tools for evaluating treatment effects, but limitations do exist. Specifically, meta-analyses require that a sufficient body of data exist to address the research question. Secondly, the population of inference and external validity of the data must be considered. These limitations are important when reviewing meta-analyses for BRD treatment and control. Insufficient data can be an issue when a meta-analysis is conducted and therapeutic options differ (eg, active drug, dose, route) from what is available currently. External validity warrants attention and the previously described meta-analyses do an excellent job of describing this limitation. When looking at BRD treatment trials in dairy-type calves, there is a limited amount of data the authors were able to identify in the literature.

The practicing clinician must make the decision to apply the results of the meta-analysis to a population of inference that may not represent their situation, identify individual trials that are more representative, or a combination thereof. A survey of producers found that preweaned heifers treated with antimicrobials for BRD are primarily treated with florfenicol (35.6%), macrolides (31.7%), and third-generation cephalosporins (10.3%).[39] When looking at weaned heifers, florfenicol, macrolides, and tetracyclines are the primary antimicrobials used for the treatment of BRD representing 31.5%, 29.1%, and 14.7%, respectively. Binversie and colleagues (2020) evaluated the effect of injectable placebo (sterile saline) or tulathromycin in 3 to 6 days of age Holstein calves diagnosed with BRD.[40] One unique aspect of this trial was the inclusion of the BRD diagnosis method (clinical presentation and ultrasound) as a blocking criterion. Treatment with tulathromycin resulted in an improvement in ADG, improvement in ultrasonographic lung scores, and lower probability of retreatment within 7 days of treatment ($P<.01$). Treatment with tulathromycin also resulted in a decrease in total mortality ($P = .05$) with 13% of the 289 calves dying before weaning compared with 22% for the placebo. For calves that survived to weaning (239 hd), similar proportions of saline (80%) and tulathromycin (81%) calves had lung consolidation ($P = .89$). The authors concluded that although antimicrobial treatment was associated with short-term benefits, more research is needed to develop treatment protocols that more effectively treat pneumonia and ensure calves enter the weaning period with ultrasonographically clean lungs. Other field trials have compared antimicrobials for the treatment of naturally occurring BRD in preweaned Holstein calves.[41,42] Researchers enrolled 696 head of Holstein heifer calves diagnosed with BRD and randomly assigned them to tulathromycin or enrofloxacin treatments. When using a multivariate logistic regression model, calves treated with enrofloxacin had 1.5 times higher odds of re-treatment 7 to 10 days after initial treatment compared with tulathromycin ($P = .04$). In addition, calves treated with enrofloxacin had 2.6 times higher odds of being treated a third time within 10 days of the second treatment compared with tulathromycin ($P = .004$). When looking at ADG, there were no statistical differences between the 2 treatments ($P = .60$). A reference in the proceedings of AABP compared Baytril (enrofloxacin) or Resflor Gold (florfenicol and flunixin meglumine) in preweaned Holstein bull calves. First-treatment success was significantly ($P<.01$) greater for Resflor Gold (50.4%) compared with Baytril (33.3%). Calves treated with Resflor Gold tended ($P = .07$) to have improved feed to gain compared with enrofloxacin.[42]

Field research trials examining the effects of BRD antimicrobial treatment on naturally occurring BRD in young dairy calves are limited. A large opportunity exists to have a more complete BRD case definition, improve BRD diagnostics, compare BRD treatment modalities, and determine lifetime impacts of BRD therapies in the young dairy animal.

BRD Control Comparisons

Similar to BRD treatment, control options have focused primarily on antimicrobial therapy. A recent meta-analysis evaluated injectable antimicrobial options for the control of BRD in the first 45 days after arrival at the feedlot.[38] In this study, it was explicitly stated that veal or dairy calves were excluded from consideration. In the absence of other data, it is tempting for a practicing clinician to use the data generated from such a large and thorough study to make BRD control decisions. For this specific meta-analysis, we know external validity is lacking because the specific population of interest (dairy calves) was excluded. It is up to the practitioner to determine the expected difference in the study population and the population of interest to see if the results are applicable to their individual practice.

Young dairy calf BRD control studies have broadly focused on administering antimicrobials in the preweaned, around the time of weaning (45–80 days of age), or long-weaned (120–180 days of age) animals. In addition, the long-acting macrolides (gamithromycin, tildipirosin, tilmicosin, and tulathromycin) have been the primary antimicrobials studied.

When reviewing studies focused on the preweaned dairy calf, the antimicrobials tildipirosin[43–45] and tulathromycin[46] have been most extensively evaluated. In a study using 1859 hd of 7 ± 7-day-old Holstein heifer calves, tildipirosin metaphylaxis significantly ($P<.01$) reduced the incidence of otitis (untreated controls = 47.03%; tildipirosin = 37.55%) and improved ADG ($P<.001$) in a 63-day period compared with untreated controls. Alternatively, Celestino (2020) and Teixeira (2017) did not see improvements in ADG compared with untreated controls. Compared with untreated controls, overall mortality tended ($P = .09$) to be improved with tildipirosin in the Bringhenti and colleagues study and with a 2-dose tildipirosin regimen in the Celenstino study ($P = .06$). Alternatively, overall mortality was not significantly different for a single dose of tildipirosin ($P = .55$) and in the Teixeira study, for either single dose or two doses of tildipirosin ($P = .11$ and $P = .21$, respectively). Stanton and colleagues (2013) found that tulathromycin-treated calves had a lower incidence of diarrhea and otitis media and increased ADG compared with calves administered an injectable placebo.[46]

BRD control studies evaluating calves around weaning have focused on the antimicrobials gamithromycin, oxytetracycline, or tulathromycin.[47–49] Linhart and Brumbaugh evaluated gamithromycin, tulathromycin, or untreated controls in a 42-day trial in dairy heifers. Gamithromycin and tulathromycin reduced treatment rates and improved ADG compared with untreated controls ($P \leq .05$). In addition, dairy heifers treated with gamithromycin had significantly ($P \leq .05$) lower BRD morbidity (34.55%) compared with tulathromycin (41.38%). No significant differences were observed for overall mortality, BRD mortality, or BRD treatment success. Stanton and colleagues (2010) evaluated tulathromycin and oxytetracycline and observed calves treated with tulathromycin were 0.5 times less likely to be treated for BRD compared with oxytetracycline. In addition, if calves had a history of BRD in the pre-enrollment period, there were no treatment differences. Alternatively, if calves had no history of BRD in the pre-enrollment period, then the oxytetracycline calves weighed 4.9 ± 0.5 kg less than the tulathromycin calves after 60 days following enrollment. When these heifer calves were followed to first calving, calves that had been treated for BRD within the first 60 days (BRD60) of the calf trial, had odds of survival 2.0 (95% confidence interval [CI], 1.1–3.6) times greater if they had received tulathromycin compared with oxytetracycline.[49] When these calves were followed to 120 days in milk, neither BRD60 nor antimicrobial treatment significantly affected survival.

When evaluating long-weaned dairy calves, a recent study evaluated gamithromycin, tildipirosin, and tulathromycin in Holstein steer calves.[50] Calves receiving gamithromycin had a lower realizer rate, lower realizer + mortality rate, and improved ribeye area at slaughter compared with tulathromycin ($P<.05$). In addition, first treatment success following metaphylaxis was significantly ($P = .02$) improved for cattle receiving gamithromycin (58.85%) compared with tulathromycin (46.85%). Economically, cattle receiving gamithromycin had a total cost of $88.54/head compared to $105.19/head for cattle receiving tulathromycin.

ANTIMICROBIAL TREATMENT AND CONTROL FAILURES

The antimicrobial treatment success or "cure" of an individual animal affected with BRD is most often determined by the clinical response in a field setting. Clinical researchers may evaluate additional response variables such as cure rate, relapse rate, ADG, lung lesions at necropsy, and mortality rate to capture meaningful data.[51] Treatment records, when available and accurate, provide practitioners key indicators of treatment failure such as case fatality rate (CFR) and retreatment rate. CFR and retreatment rate are herd-specific and may be used to monitor health trends over time to identify abnormal trends quickly. It is important to remember and understand the limited role of antimicrobials in the healing process.[52] Antimicrobials are administered to kill or inhibit the offending microbial agent assumed to be one or more bacteria in BRD cases. Therefore, if an antimicrobial fails to treat or control the disease, several factors must be considered, which may or may not be related to the drug administered.

For simplicity, non–drug-specific factors can be viewed in 1 of the following 3 categories: (1) host, (2) pathogen, and (3) administrator.[53] Essentially, factors involving one or more of the aforementioned categories may lead to treatment failures irrespective of drug selection. Examples include advanced stage of disease, pathogen virulence, compromised immune status, and concurrent disease. Drug factors contributing to perceived treatment failure are often thought to be antimicrobial resistance, which may not be fully responsible. Inaccurate case definition, poor disease detection, overdue treatment, medication errors, improper handling or storage of medicines, and others may contribute to BRD treatment failure. Lastly, antimicrobial resistance via resistance genes or mutation is of increasing concern and must be considered when BRD treatment or control failure is observed.[53]

MANAGEMENT CONSIDERATIONS

The implementation and ongoing evaluation of certain management practices tailored toward reducing disease exposure and maximizing host immunity will allow an increase in health assurance over time (**Fig. 1**).

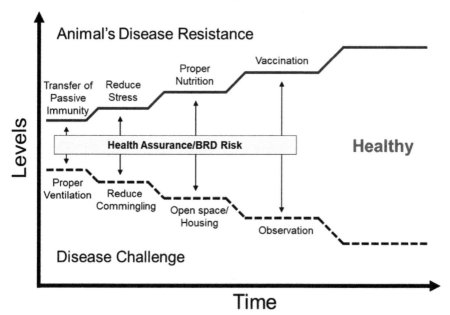

Fig. 1. (Health Assurance Spread) demonstrates the various interactions associated with increasing disease resistance and decreasing disease challenge levels over time.

A thorough on-farm assessment of the following broad areas is beneficial: calf-level and herd-level colostrum management, housing, vaccinations, nutrition, and labor. Periodic on-farm evaluations or audits prove insightful to identify areas of opportunity and should also highlight current successes.

SUMMARY

BRD affects preweaned and weaned dairy and dairy cross calves resulting in short-term and long-term losses. Practitioners must understand the etiologies and epidemiologic factors associated with BRD in young dairy calves to better assist producers in developing control and treatment strategies. When developing control and treatment protocols, practitioners should consider a thorough diagnostic approach, control and treatment strategies applicable to the population, and management opportunities to increase disease resistance and reduce disease challenge.

CLINICS CARE POINTS

- Practitioners must develop a case definition and provide training to the clinical observer for early detection of BRD.
- Routine diagnostic procedures to confirm BRD guides the practitioner when developing treatment and control strategies.
- Sound management practices and treatment/control strategies are needed for optimal BRD outcomes in young dairy calves.

DISCLOSURE

The authors have nothing to disclose.

REFERENCES

1. USDA. Dairy heifer raiser 2011. USDA-APHIS-VS, CEAH. Fort Collins (CO): National Animal Health Monitoring System (NAHMS); 2012.
2. Busby D. Tri-County Steer Carcass Futurity Data. AABP Proc 2010;43:71–81.
3. Overton MW. Economics of respiratory disease in dairy replacement heifers. Anim Health Res Rev 2020;21:143–8.
4. Woolums AR. Diseases of the Respiratory System: Lower Respiratory Tract Diseases. In: Smith BP, Van Metre DC, Pusterla N, editors. Large animal internal medicine. 6th edition. St Louis (MO): Mosby-Elsevier; 2020. p. 645–79.
5. Hughes HD, Carroll JA, Sanchez NCB, et al. Natural variations in the stress and acute phase responses of cattle. Innate Immun 2014;20(8):888–96.
6. Grissett GP, White BJ, Larson RL. Structured literature review of responses of cattle to viral and bacterial pathogens causing bovine respiratory disease complex. J Vet Intern Med 2015;29:770–80.
7. Fulton RW. Viral Diseases of the Bovine Respiratory Tract. In: Anderson DE, Rings DM, editors. Current veterinary therapy: food animal practice. 5th edition. St Louis (MO): Saunders-Elsevier; 2009. p. 171–91.
8. Ridpath J. The contribution of infections with bovine viral diarrhea viruses to bovine respiratory disease. Vet Clin North Am Food Anim Pract 2010;26:335–48.
9. Fulton RW. Viruses in bovine respiratory disease in north america: knowledge advances using genomic testing. Vet Clin North Am Food Anim Pract 2020;36:321–32.

10. Hanthorn CJ, Dewell RD, Cooper VL, et al. Randomized clinical trial to evaluate the pathogenicity of *Bibersteinia trehalosi* in respiratory disease among calves. BMC Vet Res 2014;10:89–96.

11. Maunsell FP, Woolums AR, Francoz D, et al. ACVIM Consensus Statement: *Mycoplasma bovis* Infections in Cattle. J Vet Intern Med 2011;25:772–83.

12. Rosenbusch RF. Mycoplasmas in bovine respiratory disease. In: Anderson DE, Rings DM, editors. Current veterinary therapy: food animal practice. 5th edition. St Louis (MO): Saunders-Elsevier; 2009. p. 192–4.

13. Step DL, Kirkpatrick JG. Mycoplasma infection in cattle: II. Mastitis and other diseases. Bovine Pract 2001;35(2):171–6.

14. Step DL, Confer AW, Kirkpatrick JG, et al. Respiratory tract infections in dairy calves from birth to breeding age: Detection by laboratory isolation and antibody responses. Bovine Pract 2005;39(1):44–53.

15. Virtala AK, Mechor GD, Grohn YT, et al. Epidemiologic and pathologic characteristics of respiratory tract disease in dairy heifers during the first three months of life. J Am Vet Med Assoc 1996;208(12):2035–42.

16. Clark T. *Mycoplasma bovis* – Unique Features, Pathogenesis and Lesions Update. AABP Proc 2005;38:63–6.

17. Gawthrop JC. Practitioners Experience with *Mycoplasma bovis* Outbreaks - Dairy Calves. AABP Proc 2005;38:11.

18. Lundborg GK, Svensson EC, Oltenacu PA. Herd-level risk factors for infectious diseases in Swedish dairy calves aged 0–90 days. Prev Vet Med 2005;69: 123–43.

19. Van Donkersgoed J, Ribble CS, Boyer LG, et al. Epidemiological study of enzootic pneumonia in dairy calves in Saskatchewan. Can J Vet Res 1993;57:247–54.

20. Gordon PJ, Plummer P. Control, management, and prevention of bovine respiratory disease in dairy calves and cows. Vet Clin North Am Food Anim Pract 2010; 26:243–59.

21. Griffin D. Bovine Pasteurellosis and Other Bacterial Infections of the Respiratory Tract. Vet Clin North Am Food Anim Pract 2010;26:57–71.

22. Love WJ, Lehenbauer TW, Kass PH, et al. Development of a novel clinical scoring system for on-farm diagnosis of bovine respiratory disease in pre-weaned dairy calves. PeerJ 2014;2:e238.

23. McGuirk SM, Peek SF. Timely diagnosis of dairy calf respiratory disease using a standardized scoring system. Anim Health Res Rev 2014;15:45–147.

24. McGuirk SM. Disease management of dairy calves and heifers. Vet Clin North Am Food Anim Pract 2008;24:139–53.

25. Love WJ, Lehenbauer TW, Van Eenennaam AL, et al. Sensitivity and specificity of on-farm scoring systems and nasal culture to detect bovine respiratory disease complex in preweaned dairy calves. J Vet Diagn Invest 2016;28(2):119–28.

26. Streeter RN, Step DL. Diagnostic Ultrasonography in Ruminants. Vet Clin North Am Food Anim Pract 2007;23:541–74.

27. Ollivett TL, Caswell JL, Nydam DV, et al. Thoracic ultrasonography and bronchoalveolar lavage fluid analysis in holstein calves with subclinical lung lesions. J Vet Intern Med 2015;29:1728–34.

28. Ollivett TL, Buczinkski S. On-farm use of ultrasonography for bovine respiratory disease. Vet Clin North Am Food Anim Pract 2016;32:19–35.

29. Doyle D, Credille TW, Lehenbauer R, et al. Agreement among 4 sampling methods to identify respiratory pathogens in dairy calves with acute bovine respiratory disease. J Vet Intern Med 2017;31:954–9.

30. Pardon B, Buczinski S. Bovine respiratory disease diagnosis: what progress has been made in infectious diagnosis? Vet Clin North Am Food Anim Pract 2020;36: 425–44.

31. McConnel CS, Nelson DD, Burbick CR, et al. Clarifying dairy calf mortality phenotypes through postmortem analysis. J Dairy Sci 2019;102:4415–26.

32. Severidt JA, Madden DJ, Mason GL, et al. Dairy cattle necropsy manual 2002. Available at: http://csu-cvmbs.colostate.edu/Documents/ilm-dairy-cow-necropsy-manual.pdf. April 24, 2021.

33. Step DL, Confer AW. *Mannheimia haemolytica*- and *Pasteurella multocida*-Induced Bovine Pneumonia. In: Anderson DE, Rings DM, editors. Current veterinary therapy: food animal practice. 5th edition. St Louis (MO): Saunders-Elsevier; 2009. p. 164–70.

34. American Veterinary Medical Association. Judicious therapeutic use of antimicrobials; Glossary. Schaumburg, IL, USA. 2021. Available at. https://www.avma.org/resources-tools/avma-policies/judicious-therapeutic-use-antimicrobials. May 17, 2021.

35. DeDonder KD, Apley MD. A Review of the Expected Effects of Antimicrobials in Bovine Respiratory Disease Treatment and Control Using Outcomes from Published Randomized Clinical Trials with Negative Controls. Vet Clin Food Anim 2015;31:97–111.

36. O'Connor AM, Coetzee JF, da Silva N, et al. A mixed treatment comparison meta-analysis of antibiotic treatments for bovine respiratory disease. Prev Vet Med 2013;110:77–87.

37. O'Connor AM, Yuan C, Cullen JN, et al. A mixed treatment meta-analysis of antibiotic treatment options for bovine respiratory disease – an update. Prev Vet Med 2016;132:130–9.

38. O'Connor AM, Hu D, Totton SC, et al. A systematic review and network meta-analysis of injectable antibiotic options for the control of bovine respiratory disease in the first 45 days post arrival at the feedlot. Anim Health Res Rev 2019; 20:163–81.

39. USDA. Health and management practices on U.S. Dairy operations 2014. USDA-APHIS-VS, CEAH. Fort Collins, CO: National Animal Health Monitoring System (NAHMS); 2018.

40. Binversie ES, Ruegg PL, Combs DK, et al. Randomized clinical trial to assess the effect of antibiotic therapy on health and growth of preweaned dairy calves diagnosed with respiratory disease using respiratory scoring and lung ultrasound. J Dairy Sci 2020;103:11723–35.

41. Heins BD, Nydam DV, Woolums AR, et al. Comparative efficacy of enrofloxacin and tulathromycin for treatment of preweaning respiratory disease in dairy heifers. J Dairy Sci 2014;97:372–82.

42. Sockett DC, Earleywine J, Johnson TE, et al. Performance of preweaned Holstein calves with bovine respiratory disease treated with either Resflor Gold® or Baytril®. AABP Proc 2013;46:210–1.

43. Bringhenti L, Pallu M, Silva J, et al. Effect of metaphylactic administration of tildipirosin on the incidence of pneumonia and otitis and on the upper respiratory tract and fecal microbiome of preweaning Holstein calves. J Dairy Sci 2021; 104:6020–38.

44. Celestino ML, Fernandes L, Menta PR, et al. The effect of metaphylactic use of tildipirosin for the control of respiratory disease in long-distance transported dairy calves. Front Vet Sci 2020;7:632.

45. Teixeira AGV, McArt JAA, Bicalho RC. Efficacy of tildipirosin metaphylaxis for the prevention of respiratory disease, otitis and mortality in pre-weaned Holstein calves. Vet J 2017;219:44–8.
46. Stanton AL, Kelton DF, LeBlanc SJ, et al. Effects of tulathromycin on incidence of various diseases and growth of young heifers. J Am Vet Med Assoc 2013;243: 267–76.
47. Linhart RD, Brumbaugh GW. Control of bovine respiratory disease, with and without co-morbidity by otitis media, in dairy heifers comparing gamithromycin, tulathromycin, or no medication at a commercial development facility. J Dairy Sci 2019;102:5501–10.
48. Stanton AL, Kelton DF, Leblanc SJ, et al. The effect of treatment with long-acting antibiotic at postweaning movement on respiratory disease and on growth in commercial dairy calves. J Dairy Sci 2010;93:574–81.
49. Stanton AL, Kelton DF, LeBlanc SJ, et al. The effect of respiratory disease and a preventative antibiotic treatment on growth, survival, age at first calving, and milk production of dairy heifers. J Dairy Sci 2012;95:4950–60.
50. Buchanan JW, Nilles AR, Raymond RC. Comparison of three injectable metaphylactic antimicrobial treatments administered at feedlot arrival for control of bovine respiratory disease in calf-fed Holstein steers. Bov Pract 2020;54:112–9.
51. Ollivett TL. BRD treatment failure: clinical and pathologic considerations. Anim Health Res Rev 2020;21:175–6.
52. Brumbaugh GW. The Immune System and Recovery from Sickness in Cattle. In: The Range Beef Cow Symposium XX Proceedings. 2007. Available at: https://digitalcommons.unl.edu/cgi/viewcontent.cgi?article=1015&context=rangebeef-cowsymp. April 30, 2021.
53. Booker CW, Lubbers BV. Bovine respiratory disease treatment failure: impact and potential causes. Vet Clin North Am Food Anim Pract 2020;36:487–97.

Bacterial Causes of Intestinal Disease in Dairy Calves: Acceptable Control Measures

Tamara Gull, DVM, PhD, Diplomate ACVIM(LA), ACVPM, ACVM[a],[*]

KEYWORDS

• Dairy calf • Diarrhea • *E coli* • *Salmonella* • *Clostridium perfringens* • Antibiotic

KEY POINTS

- Colibacillosis is common and best treated with supportive care (fluids, bicarbonate) until receptor loss occurs at ~7 days of age.
- Enteric salmonellosis should be treated supportively; septicemic salmonellosis requires systemic antimicrobial therapy and has a poor prognosis.
- *Clostridium perfringens* enteritis (type C or D) is uncommon in calves and is best addressed through dam vaccination and colostrum management.
- Diarrheal disease in dairy calves should not be assumed to be bacterial; laboratory testing is necessary to determine cause
- Antimicrobials should not be used empirically unless a calf is at risk of sepsis.

BACKGROUND

Bacterial causes of intestinal disease are common in calves, particularly in the neonatal period. The most common pathogens encountered are *Escherichia coli*, *Salmonella enterica*, and *Clostridium perfringens. Campylobacter* spp. have also been occasionally implicated. Although calf diarrhea is unlikely to be able to be completely eliminated from a herd, a goal should be to have less than 3% death losses from diarrhea. This goal can be achieved through appropriate herd management and targeted treatment of affected calves.

PATHOGENESIS

Bacteria contribute to the pathogenesis of calf diarrhea primarily through stimulation of increased secretion from enterocytes; this is often induced, for instance, in

[a] Bacteriology/Mycology, U.S. Army Veterinary Corps
[*] Veterinary Medical Diagnostic Laboratory, University of Missouri CVM, 901 E. Campus Loop, Columbia, MO 65211.
E-mail address: tgull@missouri.edu

Vet Clin Food Anim 38 (2022) 107–119
https://doi.org/10.1016/j.cvfa.2021.11.008
0749-0720/22/© 2021 Elsevier Inc. All rights reserved.

enterotoxigenic *E coli* (ETEC), via secretion of toxins that activate cyclic adenosine monophosphate, cyclic guanine monophosphate, calmodulin, or tyrosine kinase.[1–3] The cell's structure is generally not affected in these cases. Other organisms (eg, *Salmonella*, enteropathogenic *E. coli*) may secrete cytotoxins that directly damage the intestinal epithelial cells.[4] In general, bacteria induce the loss of bicarbonate, electrolytes, and water. Bicarbonate loss contributes to acidosis along with increased L-lactate synthesis from poor perfusion secondary to dehydration. D-lactate synthesis by bacteria further worsens acidosis.

Escherichia coli (colibacillosis)

Diarrhea caused by *E. coli* is the most common bacterial cause of calf diarrhea. There are many strains of *E. coli*, and most are nonpathogenic normal flora. A small number of *E. coli* strains are considered pathogenic and can cause diarrhea. ETEC is seen only in neonatal calves, usually in the first 4 days of life, but colibacillosis caused by other types of *E. coli* can occur in older calves. Colibacillosis pathogenesis first requires adherence of the bacteria to the intestinal epithelium via fimbrial (pilus) antigens, and then expression of toxin to create the pathogenic effects. ETEC do not produce any gross or histologic lesions because the toxins induce hypersecretion but do not physically damage enterocytes. ETEC produce fimbrial antigens, most commonly F5(K99), and secrete enterotoxins, primarily the heat-stable enterotoxin STa although other fimbrial antigens and toxins may be expressed. The receptors to which the ETEC fimbriae bind cease expression by approximately a week of age. Diarrhea induced by ETEC is not hemorrhagic.

Diarrhea in older calves may be caused by *E. coli* of the attaching and effacing (AEEC), Shiga-toxin-producing (STEC), or enteropathogenic (EPEC) types. In these types of colibacillosis, unlike in ETEC, there is histologically visible damage to the intestine. Non-ETEC diarrhea outbreaks have been documented in calves from 2 days to 4 weeks of age, and non-ETEC pathogenic isolates have been detected at higher frequency in diarrheic calves, although pathogenic *E. coli* may also be found in nondiarrheic animals.[5] The actual link between AEEC/STEC/EPEC and nonneonatal bovine diarrhea is still poorly elucidated because most laboratories do not routinely type fecal *E. coli*.

The Shiga-toxin-producing enterohemorrhagic *E. coli* (STEC/EHEC) implicated in human hemorrhagic colitis and pediatric hemolytic-uremic syndrome is usually associated with serotype O157. This serotype is commonly found in calf feces[6] but is not considered pathogenic in the bovine and has rarely been implicated as a cause of calf diarrhea.[7] This serotype is a potential zoonotic risk, and control measures may be warranted depending on the production goals of the dairy.

Salmonella

Salmonella enterica is another common bacterial cause of calf diarrhea and can affect cattle of any age. Most enteric salmonellosis in cattle is caused by *S. enterica* serotype Typhimurium or serotype Dublin, although other serotypes have been isolated. *S.* Dublin is considered host-adapted to cattle, meaning that a true carrier state exists and the disease is often endemic in herds. *S.* Dublin uncommonly causes clinical disease in adult cattle, but asymptomatic carriers may transmit the organism to calves that subsequently become clinically ill.[8,9] In contrast, the disease caused by non-host-adapted *S.* Typhimurium commonly manifests as epidemic, resulting in morbidity in all ages of cattle. It is important to identify the serotype because control measures differ.

Disease caused by *Salmonella* is more common in younger calves because the infective dose necessary to induce disease increases with calf age.[10,11] Calves are commonly subjected to significant *Salmonella* challenge in the first days of life, because the organism can be shed in large numbers in feces and milk and may even be transmitted *in utero*.[12] Premises sanitation plays a large role in *Salmonella* diarrhea, because shedding occurs via any secretion and can persist on bottles, nipples, buckets, esophageal feeders, medicating utensils, and wet manure packs; environmental *Salmonella* can exceed the infective dose threshold.

Salmonella preferentially affects the distal small intestine and proximal large bowel, although lesions can occur in any part of the gastrointestinal (GI) tract. Histologically, fibrinous to necrotic ulcerative enteritis is seen, often with dysentery. Mesenteric lymphadenopathy is common. Pneumonia is often encountered with *S*. Dublin, and septic infarcts can be seen in many tissues.

Clostridium perfringens

Clostridial species are a less common sporadic bacterial cause of calf diarrhea, and determining that these organisms are causative is difficult. *C. perfringens* is a normal inhabitant of the bovine intestinal tract, and all *C. perfringens* have the potential to secrete various enterotoxins. The specific toxins encoded in the genome determine the type of *C. perfringens* present; type A through type E are considered relevant in livestock. The presence of a toxin gene does not, however, prove that the toxins are being secreted. Linking *C. perfringens* with disease requires the presence of characteristic clinical signs or necropsy lesions along with evidence of the presence of toxin.[13–15] Most laboratories do not routinely type *C. perfringens* isolates, and even fewer have the ability to perform toxin assays. *C. perfringens* type A is commonly isolated from feces of both healthy and diarrheic animals, whereas types B to E are less commonly isolated.[13] Type A is associated with acute hemorrhagic abomasitis in neonates that manifests as colic, abdominal distention, depression, and death. Necropsy lesions include abomasitis, abomasal ulcers, and abomasal tympany. Type A-linked hemorrhagic enteritis may also be seen in older (2- to 4-month) calves with similar clinical signs. Necropsy lesions include hemorrhagic and necrotic enteritis of the small intestine.

C. perfringens type C produces alpha and beta toxin. Beta toxin is susceptible to trypsin degradation, and disease is most commonly seen in neonates younger than 10 days; this reflects the trypsin inhibitors present in the intestine of the young calf.[16] Clinical signs in these young calves include abdominal pain and neurologic signs, but sudden death may also occur. Necropsy reveals hemorrhagic and necrotic enteritis.[16] *C. perfringens* types D and E have been infrequently reported as a cause of hemorrhagic enteritis and abomasitis in calves.[17,18]

Clostridioides (formerly *Clostridium*) *difficile* has been isolated from both healthy and diarrheic calves but has not been specifically linked to disease.[19–21]

Campylobacter spp.

Whether *Campylobacter* spp. cause diarrhea in calves is undetermined at this point because both *Campylobacter jejuni* and *Campylobacter coli* have been isolated from both normal and diarrheic calves with approximately equal frequency.[22] Enteritis can be induced through administration of *C. jejuni* or *C. coli,* both organisms that have been associated with diarrheal disease in other species.[23]

EVALUATION

The adverse effects of diarrhea in calves are most commonly attributed to fluid loss, electrolyte and acid-base imbalance, and secondary septicemia. Evaluation of the diarrheic calf should focus on these aspects of the calf's condition, because the severity of clinical signs can guide both selected treatment and prognosis. Assessment should include a complete physical examination, nutrition assessment, and fecal evaluation. Particular attention should be paid to temperature, hydration status and suckle behavior, attitude, and whether signs of extraintestinal disease are present. The presence of significant extraintestinal disease (eg, joint effusion, hypopyon, meningitis) is a poor prognostic indicator. Hydration assessment in acute diarrhea is best done by the degree of enophthalmos, whereas cervical skin tent is better in cases of chronic diarrhea. Ancillary testing such as pen-side acid-base, electrolyte, or lactate measurement is helpful.

Many diagnostic laboratories offer an enteric panel that evaluates the presence of bacterial, viral, protozoal, and parasitic pathogens. At least 25 g/25 mL of feces should be submitted to the diagnostic laboratory for these panels, and specimens for culture should be immediately shipped overnight with cold packs whenever possible. In addition, larger sample volumes improve the odds of successfully culturing relevant bacteria. Fecal swabs are of insufficient quantity for most panels. In mortality cases, either the entire carcass or a selection of fresh and formalin-fixed enteric tissues should be submitted. Samples collected must be fresh because autolysis and alterations in bacterial flora start within minutes of death. Ideally samples would be collected from animals early in disease and before any treatments have been instituted. Fresh feces or tissue should be packaged in such a way as to exclude air from the specimen to optimize anaerobe recovery; Whirl-Paks (Madison, WI, USA) are excellent for this purpose because air can be squeezed out of the bag before it is sealed. Standard zipper-closure plastic bags and palpation sleeves or examination gloves are not appropriate containers because of leakage and laboratory worker safety concerns. If cups are used they should be filled to the brim to exclude air. If overnight shipping of samples is not possible, submission of fecal swabs in transport media may allow recovery of pathogens. Swabs such as those using at least 1 mL of liquid transport medium (eg, ESwabs) will maintain nonfastidious anaerobes well. Culture of fastidious anaerobes such as C. difficile is challenging, and diagnosis may be more appropriately achieved via toxin detection. A veterinary microbiologist can advise on appropriate collection and handling of culture specimens if a specific pathogen is being sought.

Diagnosis of diarrhea attributable to E. coli first requires culturing the organism from feces or tissue. Any veterinary diagnostic laboratory would be able to do the basic culture. Typing of the E. coli can determine whether it is pathogenic (ETEC, EPEC/AEEC/STEC, etc.); typing is available only at a few laboratories. The diagnostic laboratory that does the routine culture can forward a pure culture of the isolate to a typing laboratory upon request. Once the type is known, this information can be used to determine if the type isolated correlates with the clinical signs and/or necropsy lesions. A veterinary pathologist can assist with evaluation of necropsy lesions in correlation with the typing results. Judicious use principles for antimicrobials indicate that cultured E. coli should not be treated unless typing indicates a potential pathogen and clinical signs/necropsy lesions are supportive.

Diagnosis of disease attributable to Salmonella requires isolation of the organism from feces or tissue. Most diagnostic laboratories are equipped to do this, but it is appropriate to specifically request Salmonella culture because it requires additional enrichment and the use of selective media. If the laboratory does not routinely do so, the submitter should request that any Salmonella isolate be serotyped because this can guide control principles. Polymerase chain reaction of feces or tissue for Salmonella is also widely available and may be faster than culture, but this does not yield a serotype. Isolation of Salmonella from feces alone does not indicate causation, because *Salmonella* can be isolated from normal calves. Fecal identification of *Salmonella* should be confirmed as the cause of disease through visualization of appropriate necropsy lesions. Isolation of *Salmonella* from extraintestinal tissues is confirmatory of the diagnosis.

Diagnosis of diarrhea caused by *Clostridium* species can be challenging due to the fastidiousness of the organisms and the difficulty in linking organism isolation with the ability to cause disease. One of the more useful tools for diagnosis of clostridial enteritis is histopathologic examination of fresh necropsy intestinal tissue; visualization of large numbers of Gram-positive rods in association with hemorrhagic enteritis is suggestive. If organism isolation is desired, anaerobic culture from a sample held in conditions that support the maintenance of anaerobic organisms is necessary. Genotyping of *C. perfringens* is necessary to determine potential pathogenicity, but this information must be considered along with the lesions present before causation can be assessed. Ideally, immunoassay or Western blot could be used to detect toxin production, but these tests are not widely available and are technically difficult.

THERAPEUTIC OPTIONS

Treatment of diarrheal disease in calves should have 4 goals: correction of dehydration and electrolyte abnormalities, correction of acid-base abnormalities, provision of nutrition; and last, treatment of bacterial infection. Fluid therapy should be oral whenever possible, but intravenous fluids may be necessary for very sick calves. Oral rehydration solutions are widely commercially available. An appropriate solution for a diarrheic calf should include 90 to 130 mmol/L sodium, 40 to 80 mEq/L chloride, and 10 to 30 mmol/L potassium and should have an osmolality of 300 to 600 mOsm. Oral rehydration solutions intended to treat diarrhea should also contain an alkalinizing agent (acetate, propionate, bicarbonate, or citrate) at greater than 50 mmol/L. These solutions should have a strong ion difference of greater than 60; strong ion difference can be calculated as [Na] +[K]−[Cl]. Glucose will be present in these solutions and is the primary determinant of osmolality.

In flat, weak calves for which oral rehydration is not appropriate, intravenous fluid support should be instituted. Fluid deficit in liters should be estimated as percent dehydration × body weight in kilograms. Ongoing losses should also be estimated and added to the deficit, as should daily maintenance of 50 to 100 mL/kg/d. As diarrheic calves are typically acidotic, alkalinizing fluids such as 0.9% saline or Ringer's are recommended. Calves may also benefit from exogenous bicarbonate administration. If bicarbonate or total CO_2 measurement is available, bicarbonate deficit may be calculated as body weight(kg) × base deficit (equal to 30 − bicarbonate measurement or TCO_2 in mmol/L) × 0.6. The bicarbonate deficit may be administered as isotonic bicarbonate or diluted into saline or Ringer's, and the deficit should be corrected within 24 hours. Ongoing diarrhea will generate ongoing deficits that must be taken into account. If measurement of bicarbonate or TCO_2 is not available, bicarbonate deficits may be estimated: in a standing calf, 250 mmol HCO_3 may be administered, whereas in a weak calf that is able to stand 500 mmol may be used. In recumbent calves, 750 mmol of bicarbonate may be given. Isotonic bicarbonate solutions (156 mmol/L) can be mixed by dissolving 13 g baking soda in 1 L water. Fluids should be warmed before administration if the calf is hypothermic. Bicarbonate should not be added to calcium-containing fluids.

Nutrition is also important in the diarrheic calf, and oral rehydration solutions do not provide sufficient glucose to meet nutritional needs, although some "high-energy" rehydration solutions may be able to provide 50% to 75% of caloric requirements. Whole milk is a better option for nutrition whenever possible, and most inappetent calves will regain appetite once electrolyte therapy has been instituted. Milk withdrawal of ~12 hours may be considered in the inappetent calf, but longer milk withdrawals may result in cachexia. Milk feeding is best done on a voluntary basis by nipple bottle or bucket, because tube feeding may result in pooling of milk in the reticulorumen. Calf starter or roughage should be available for older calves.

The final aspect of treatment in diarrheal disease of calves is antimicrobial therapy. Although antibiotics are often thought of as first-line therapies for bacterial disease, most calves with diarrhea do not require antimicrobial therapy. Systemic antimicrobials may be suboptimal for use in enteric disease for several reasons. First, normal flora is further disrupted. Second, few antimicrobials are labeled for use in bovine enteric disease and withdrawal times may not be well established. Third, an increasing body of evidence demonstrates that use of antimicrobials on a farm (for any purpose) induces resistance in enteric flora even if no antimicrobials have been used specifically to treat enteric disease, further decreasing the available options. The administration of antimicrobials specifically to calves has been identified as one of the major drivers of antimicrobial resistance on a farm. Although antimicrobials may be considered as therapy for an individual calf, antimicrobial prophylaxis or metaphylaxis of a group of calves for enteric disease is not recommended and does not improve mortality. Prophylactic feeding of antimicrobials to calves is now illegal in many countries because of its effects on antimicrobial resistance. Instead, preventive measures such as colostrum management, vaccination, sanitation, and biosecurity are of high importance in calf-rearing operations.

When antimicrobial therapy is considered, determination of the causative agent is necessary before the initiation of therapy; this is particularly true given that nonbacterial causes of diarrhea are extremely common in calves and antimicrobial therapy is both ineffective and potentially resistance generating in nonbacterial enteric disease. Also, whereas confirmation of the causative organism is necessary, susceptibility determination is not. Calves can routinely carry multiple strains of E. coli, and the strain of an organism isolated from feces is often different from the strain present at the site of infection in the small intestine. Instead, general treatment recommendations targeted toward E. coli and Salmonella have been propagated. These recommended drugs may not be labeled for the treatment of diarrhea in cattle, and withdrawals have not been established. Consultation with the Food Animal Residue Avoidance Databank (FARAD; www.farad.org) is strongly recommended.

For calves in which bacterial diarrhea has been confirmed, recommended antimicrobial therapy depends on the calf's status. Diarrheic calves with no fever that are still eating do not require antimicrobial therapy. Preruminating calves that are ill but not suspect for bacteremia may be treated with oral antimicrobials. Amoxicillin trihydrate at 10 mg/kg by mouth twice a day reduces the duration of diarrhea and mortality[24,25]; this drug may be combined with clavulanate for increased efficacy. Sulfadiazine at 25 mg/kg combined with trimethoprim at 5 mg/kg by mouth daily for 5 days reduced Salmonella mortality in an experimental study.[26] Apramycin at 20 to 40 mg/kg by mouth daily for 5 days reduced both mortality and duration of diarrhea in another study.[27] Apramycin and other aminoglycosides are not absorbed from the GI tract, making them appropriate choices for ETEC infections only.

Calves that are severely ill with greater than 6% dehydration, recumbency, and depression or otherwise deemed at risk for septicemia should receive parenteral antimicrobial therapy. Protocols that have shown efficacy include trimethoprim/sulfadiazine (5 mg/kg/25 mg/kg subcutaneously daily) in 2- to 3-week-old calves[28]; serum trimethoprim concentrations decrease rapidly in older calves, and sulfadiazine is ineffective as a solo medication. Amoxicillin at 11 to 15 mg/kg intramuscularly (IM) once daily reduced mortality in *S.* Dublin-infected calves,[29] and ampicillin trihydrate at 22 mg/kg SQ or IM once daily reduced mortality in naturally occurring diarrhea.[30] Florfenicol at 20 mg/kg IM every 48 hours for 2 doses has shown efficacy against *Salmonella*.[31] Ceftiofur hydrochloride at 5 mg/kg IM for 5 days reduced clinical signs and fecal shedding of *Salmonella*.[32] It should be emphasized that third-generation cephalosporins and cephamycins (such as ceftiofur) are considered critically important human drugs by the World Health Organization and should not be used in animals until other antimicrobials are demonstrated to be ineffective. In the United States, cephalosporins may be used for extralabel indications but must be used in accordance with label dose, route, frequency, and duration. The 5 mg/kg ceftiofur dose in the abovementioned paper is not in compliance with the US label and would not be permitted in the United States. It must also be emphasized that fluoroquinolones (e.g. enrofloxacin and danofloxacin) are prohibited from extralabel use in the United States and may never be used in the treatment of diarrheal disease in cattle.

There are no specific studies investigating antimicrobial use in calf diarrhea caused by *Clostridium* spp. If clostridial organisms are confirmed as the cause of diarrheal disease, best practices would suggest administration of a β-lactam drug such as oral amoxicillin in preruminating calves and injectable amoxicillin or ampicillin in older calves.

ANCILLARY TREATMENTS

Anti-inflammatory drugs should be administered to systemically ill calves once fluid support has ensured appropriate renal output. Meloxicam given at 0.5 mg/kg SQ or IV once increased feed consumption, improved diarrhea, and decreased signs of colic.[33] Flunixin meglumine at 2.2 mg/kg IM may also improve morbidity.[34] No more than 3 once-daily doses of either should be given to avoid abomasal mucosal damage. Corticosteroids are not recommended. There is no evidence supporting the use of bismuth subsalicylate, ketoprofen, or aspirin.[35] Probiotics and prebiotics have been investigated as an alternative to antimicrobials in the treatment of bacterial diarrhea; neither have been demonstrated to be effective treatments, although they may have a role in diarrhea prevention.[36–38] Lactoferrin, which is naturally found in colostrum, may show promise as a nonantibiotic therapy. One study investigating lactoferrin reported a decrease in mortality and a lowered risk of culling by 60 days in calves that were severely diarrheic, but another study showed no benefit on mortality.[39,40]

PREVENTION

Prevention of disease is always better than treatment. In infectious disease, prevention relies on several factors including minimizing exposure, ensuring adequate colostrum feeding, enhancing immunity, and maintaining biosecurity. Minimizing exposure is achieved through sanitation and segregation. First, cows should calve in a clean environment separate from other animals; calving pens should never be used as sick pens. Calving pens should be completely cleaned and disinfected between cows. The external genitalia and udder of cows should be washed before calving. Milk fed to calves should be of high quality and should be pasteurized before feeding; waste milk or milk containing antibiotic residues should not be fed to calves. Acidified milk or replacer may decrease nonspecific diarrheal disease.[41,42] Milk for calves should be kept refrigerated to inhibit bacterial growth and warmed just before feeding. Milk replacer, if fed, should be mixed using a clean water source, and feeding equipment should be scrubbed with soap and disinfected after each use; rinsing alone is ineffective. A standard kitchen dishwasher can be helpful. Bags of milk replacer should be stored closed and protected from contamination, and scoops should be regularly disinfected. Personnel should adhere to strict hand hygiene before and during mixing and feeding.

Dairy calves should not be raised in groups because this increases the risk of diarrhea.[43] Calf hutches, if used, should be thoroughly cleaned and disinfected between occupants; physical scrubbing is necessary. Pressure washing is discouraged because this can aerosolize pathogens and promote spread. Concrete pads should be disinfected after cleaning and left exposed to sunlight for several days. Waste left behind when a hutch is moved should be picked up and disposed of, and the ground raked and left exposed for several sunny days. Clean hutches should be sited on ground or pads not recently used. Cleaner and disinfectant use must strictly adhere to label instructions, particularly with mixing instructions and contact time. A multipurpose disinfectant such as a peroxygen or other oxidizing agent is generally effective against all common pathogens except *Cryptosporidium* when used according to label instructions.

Colostrum management is of extreme importance, particularly in the prevention of ETEC diarrhea. Colostrum contains antibodies that bind to the bacterial fimbriae in the intestinal lumen and prevent adherence to intestinal epithelial cells; without adherence, the bacteria are unable to colonize the intestine and cause disease. This effect of colostrum is separate from passive transfer, as IgG in serum is ineffective at preventing intestinal *E. coli* colonization. Thus even calves with measured failure of passive transfer may still be protected against *E. coli* colonization if sufficient antibody is present in the intestinal lumen. However, as with any bacteria, the number of bacteria present may overwhelm the amount of antibody, further emphasizing the importance of sanitation in decreasing the environmental bacterial burden. The udder and surrounding areas should be cleaned and disinfected when collecting colostrum from cows and the colostrum should be heat treated if possible (60°C for 30–60 minutes). Colostrum replacers should be used if colostrum is not available but may not be as effective. Additional colostrum feedings may help in decreasing diarrhea incidence.[44]

Dam vaccination is a recommended method for boosting immunity and decreasing calf diarrhea due to bacterial pathogens.[45,46] As ETEC is seen early in life, calves have insufficient time to mount an endogenous immune response. However, dam vaccination can result in colostrum containing high levels of specific antibody. ETEC vaccines directed against F5(K99) are recommended at 6 and 3 weeks before calving; ensuring appropriate colostral intake is, of course, necessary.

There are several *Salmonella* vaccine products available, both bacterins and modified live. In general, the modified live vaccines demonstrate better efficacy.[47–49] Calves immunized with modified live vaccines showed protection against both homologous and heterologous challenges in short-term studies.[50,51] The *Salmonella* vaccines are not specifically designed for colostral protection and any such protection is likely short-lived; however, dam vaccination may be of benefit on farms with endemic salmonellosis. For ongoing benefit, both calves and cows should be vaccinated. No clostridial vaccines are specifically labeled for prevention of calf diarrhea. However, there are reports of decreased calf diarrhea incidence in herds vaccinated with multivalent clostridial products and neutralizing antibodies can be generated.[52]

Nonspecific immunity relies on several factors. Diet is important, because the calf cannot respond to infectious challenge without appropriate nutrition. When calves are fed limited amounts of milk replacer daily their nutritional needs rapidly outpace the nutrition available via milk or milk replacer. The calf then must make up the deficit through consumption of calf starter. Delays in the calf consuming starter can result in a stressed calf that is more susceptible to infectious disease. To prevent this, a high-quality starter must be provided and unconsumed starter should be disposed of daily and the feeding bucket cleaned and disinfected. Starter consumption should be monitored and lack of consumption investigated. Other nonpharmaceutical means have also been suggested to improve calf health and prevent diarrhea. Administration of vitamin A supplementation and feeding of yeast fermentation products have been suggested, with variable efficacy.[53–55] Probiotics, which contain nonpathogenic intestinal organisms, have also been suggested in the prevention of diarrhea. There is some evidence that probiotics may reduce the incidence, duration, or severity of bacterial diarrhea when administered before challenge. The probiotics that have demonstrated these effects contained a mixture of lactic acid bacteria (eg, *Lactobacillus, Streptococcus, Enterococcus*), *E. coli* strain Nissle 1917, or *Faecalibacterium prausnitzii*.[36,37,56] In contrast, prebiotics have not been demonstrated to have any beneficial effect on the incidence of bacterial diarrhea.[57] Supplementation of zinc may be beneficial in the prevention of nonspecific diarrhea,[58,59] as may administration of egg yolk (IgY) antibody products.[60]

Biosecurity is maintained through careful selection of replacement animals. Replacements should be purchased directly from a single farm of origin, if possible, and as few sources as practical if not. Purchase of animals from multiple sources and auction houses is a risk factor for the acquisition of infectious disease along with the new animals. Cows identified as carriers of *S. Dublin* via repeated milk or colostral culture may be considered for culling because they represent an ongoing biosecurity threat.

SUMMARY

Bacterial diarrhea is common in calves but must be distinguished from enteric disease caused by other organisms to facilitate optimal treatment. Accurate diagnosis requires laboratory testing of appropriately collected samples. Antibiotics should not be used as empirical therapy for diarrhea unless sepsis is suspected, but fluid and electrolyte support is vital. Incidence of bacterial diarrhea can be decreased through appropriate herd interventions.

CLINICS CARE POINTS

- Maintain a vaccination program for bacterial pathogens, and ensure every calf receives colostrum or colostrum replacer.
- Maintain sanitary calving pens, and do not use calving pens as sick pens.
- Obtain an accurate etiologic diagnosis through physical examination, necropsy, and laboratory testing.
- Intervene early in the diarrheal disease process with fluid and electrolyte/bicarbonate support.
- Do not use antibiotics as first-line treatment; use only when bacterial pathogens are confirmed.
- Know what bacterial pathogens are present on the farm and adjust the vaccination, sanitation, and culling of animals accordingly

DISCLOSURE

The author has nothing to disclose.

REFERENCES

1. Acres SD. Enterotoxigenic Escherichia coli infections in newborn calves: a review. J Dairy Sci 1985;68(1):229–56.
2. Argenzio RA. Pathophysiology of neonatal calf diarrhea. Vet Clin North Am Food Anim Pract 1985;1(3):461–9.
3. Foster DM, Smith GW. Pathophysiology of diarrhea in calves. Vet Clin North Am Food Anim Pract 2009;25(1):13–36, xi.
4. Zhang S, Santos RL, Tsolis RM, et al. The Salmonella enterica serotype Typhimurium effector proteins SipA, SopA, SopB, SopD, and SopE2 act in concert to induce diarrhea in calves. Infect Immun 2002;70(7):3843–55.
5. de Moura C, Ludovico M, Valadares GF, et al. Detection of virulence genes in Escherichia coli strains isolated from diarrheic and healthy feces of dairy calves in Brazil. Arq Inst Biol (São Paulo) 2012;79(2):273–6.
6. Engelen F, Thiry D, Devleesschauwer B, et al. Pathogenic potential of Escherichia coli O157 and O26 isolated from young Belgian dairy calves by recto-anal mucosal swab culturing. J Appl Microbiol 2021;131(2):964–72.
7. Awad WS, El-Sayed AA, Mohammed FF, et al. Molecular characterization of pathogenic Escherichia coli isolated from diarrheic and in-contact cattle and buffalo calves. Trop Anim Health Prod 2020;52(6):3173–85.
8. Richardson A. The transmission of Salmonella Dublin to calves from adult carrier cows. Vet Rec 1973;92(5):112–5.
9. Smith BP, Oliver DG, Singh P, et al. Detection of Salmonella Dublin mammary gland infection in carrier cows, using an enzyme-linked immunosorbent assay for antibody in milk or serum. Am J Vet Res 1989;50(8):1352–60.
10. Snider TA, Gull T, Jackson TA, et al. Experimental salmonellosis challenge model in older calves. Vet Microbiol 2014;170(1–2):65–72.
11. Rankin JD, Taylor RJ. The estimation of doses of Salmonella Typhimurium suitable for the experimental production of disease in calves. Vet Rec 1966;78(21):706–7.
12. Hanson DL, Loneragan GH, Brown TR, et al. Evidence supporting vertical transmission of Salmonella in dairy cattle. Epidemiol Infect 2016;144(5):962–7.
13. Ferrarezi MC, Cardoso TC, Dutra IS. Genotyping of Clostridium perfringens isolated from calves with neonatal diarrhea. Anaerobe 2008;14(6):328–31.
14. Lozano EA, Catlin JE, Hawkins WW. Incidence of Clostridium perfringens in neonatal enteritis of Montana calves. Cornell Vet 1970;60(3):347–59.
15. Len'kov VI, Len'kova VA, Iakubo EP. [Diagnosis of enterotoxemia of calves caused by Clostridium perfringens]. Veterinariia 1966;43(4):30–1.
16. Griner LA, Bracken FK. Clostridium perfringens (type C) in acute hemorrhagic enteritis of calves. J Am Vet Med Assoc 1953;122(911):99–102.
17. Songer JG, Miskimmins DW. Clostridium perfringens type E enteritis in calves: two cases and a brief review of the literature. Anaerobe 2004;10(4):239–42.
18. Watson PJ, Scholes SF. Clostridium perfringens type D epsilon intoxication in one-day-old calves. Vet Rec 2009;164(26):816–7.
19. Rodriguez-Palacios A, Stämpfli HR, Duffield T, et al. Clostridium difficile PCR ribotypes in calves, Canada. Emerg Infect Dis 2006;12(11):1730–6.
20. Magistrali CF, Maresca C, Cucco L, et al. Prevalence and risk factors associated with Clostridium difficile shedding in veal calves in Italy. Anaerobe 2015;33:42–7.

21. Houser BA, Soehnlen MK, Wolfgang DR, et al. Prevalence of Clostridium difficile toxin genes in the feces of veal calves and incidence of ground veal contamination. Foodborne Pathog Dis 2012;9(1):32–6.
22. Adesiyun AA, Kaminjolo JS, Loregnard R, et al. Campylobacter infections in calves, piglets, lambs and kids in Trinidad. Br Vet J 1992;148(6):547–56.
23. Warner DP, Bryner JH. Campylobacter jejuni and Campylobacter coli inoculation of neonatal calves. Am J Vet Res 1984;45(9):1822–4.
24. Palmer GH, Bywater RJ, Francis ME. Amoxycillin: distribution and clinical efficacy in calves. Vet Rec 1977;100(23):487–91.
25. RJ B. Evaluation of an oral glucose-glycine-electrolyte formulation and amoxicillin for treatment of diarrhea in calves. Am J Vet Res 1977;38:1983.
26. White G, Pearcy D, Gibbs HA. Use of a calf salmonellosis model to evaluate the therapeutic properties of trimethoprim and sulfadiazine and their mutual potentiation in vivo. Res Vet Sci 1981;31(27):27–31.
27. Pankhurst JW, D.M., Zeri A. The treatment of disease in the young calf with apramycin. in 20th World Veterinary Congress. 1975. Thessaloniki Greece.
28. Daniels LB, Fineberg D, Cockrill JM, et al. Use of trimethoprim-sulfadiazine in controlling calf scours. Vet Med Small Anim Clin 1977;72(1):93–5.
29. Osborne AD, Nazer AH, Shimeld C. Treatment of experimental calf salmonellosis with amoxycillin. Vet Rec 1978;103(11):233–7.
30. Grimshaw WT, Colman PJ, Petrie L. Efficacy of sulbactam-ampicillin in the treatment of neonatal calf diarrhoea. Vet Rec 1987;121(8):162–6.
31. Silva DG, Silva PRL, S.P, Fagliari JJ. Efficacy of florfenicol and intravenous fluid therapy for treatment of experimental salmonellosis in newborn calves. Arq Bras Med Vet Zootec 2010;(62):499–503.
32. Fecteau M-E, House JK, Kotarski SF, et al. Efficacy of ceftiofur for treatment of experimental salmonellosis in neonatal calves. Am J Vet Res 2003;64(7):918–25.
33. Philipp H, Schmidt H, Düring F, et al. Efficacy of meloxicam (Metacam®) as adjunct to a basic therapy for the treatment of diarrhoea in calves. Acta Veterinaria Scand Supplementum 2003;(No.supp. 98):273.
34. Barnett SC, Sischo WM, Moore DA, et al. Evaluation of flunixin meglumine as an adjunct treatment for diarrhea in dairy calves. J Am Vet Med Assoc 2003;223(9): 1329–33.
35. Berge ACB, Lindeque P, Moore DA, et al. A clinical trial evaluating prophylactic and therapeutic antibiotic use on health and performance of preweaned calves. J Dairy Sci 2005;88(6):2166–77.
36. Signorini ML, Soto LP, Zbrun MV, et al. Impact of probiotic administration on the health and fecal microbiota of young calves: a meta-analysis of randomized controlled trials of lactic acid bacteria. Res Vet Sci 2012;93(1):250–8.
37. Uyeno Y, Shigemori S, Shimosato T. Effect of Probiotics/Prebiotics on Cattle Health and Productivity. Microbes Environ 2015;30(2):126–32.
38. Renaud DL, Kelton DF, Weese JS, et al. Evaluation of a multispecies probiotic as a supportive treatment for diarrhea in dairy calves: A randomized clinical trial. J Dairy Sci 2019;102(5):4498–505.
39. Habing G, Harris K, Schuenemann GM, et al. Lactoferrin reduces mortality in preweaned calves with diarrhea. J Dairy Sci 2017;100(5):3940–8.
40. Pempek JA, Watkins LR, Bruner CE, et al. A multisite, randomized field trial to evaluate the influence of lactoferrin on the morbidity and mortality of dairy calves with diarrhea. J Dairy Sci 2019;102(10):9259–67.

41. Li L, Qu J, Xin X, et al. Comparison of reconstituted, acidified reconstituted milk or acidified fresh milk on growth performance, diarrhea rate, and hematological parameters in preweaning dairy calves. Animals (Basel) 2019;9(10):778.
42. Zou Y, Wang Y, Deng Y, et al. Effects of feeding untreated, pasteurized and acidified waste milk and bunk tank milk on the performance, serum metabolic profiles, immunity, and intestinal development in Holstein calves. J Anim Sci Biotechnol 2017;8:53.
43. Losinger WC, Heinrichs AJ. Management practices associated with high mortality among preweaned dairy heifers. J Dairy Res 1997;64(1):1–11.
44. Kargar S, Roshan M, Ghoreishi SM, et al. Extended colostrum feeding for 2 weeks improves growth performance and reduces the susceptibility to diarrhea and pneumonia in neonatal Holstein dairy calves. J Dairy Sci 2020;103(9):8130–42.
45. Collins NF, Halbur T, Schwenck WH, et al. Duration of immunity and efficacy of an oil emulsion Escherichia coli bacterin in cattle. Am J Vet Res 1988;49(5):674–7.
46. Valente C, Fruganti G, Tesei B, et al. Vaccination of pregnant cows with K99 antigen of enterotoxigenic Escherichia coli and protection by colostrum in newborn calves. Comp Immunol Microbiol Infect Dis 1988;11(3–4):189–98.
47. Aitken MM, Jones PW, Brown GT. Protection of cattle against experimentally induced salmonellosis by intradermal injection of heat-killed Salmonella Dublin. Res Vet Sci 1982;32(3):368–73.
48. Baljer G, Hoerstke M, Dirksen G, et al. [Comparative studies of the effectivity of oral immunization with heat-inactivated and live, avirulent (Gal E-) S. Typhimurium bacteria against salmonellosis in calves]. Zentralbl Veterinarmed B 1981; 28(9–10):759–66.
49. Jones PW, Dougan G, Hayward N, et al. Oral vaccination of calves against experimental salmonellosis using a double aro mutant of Salmonella Typhimurium. Vaccine 1991;9(1):29–34.
50. Rankin JD, Taylor RJ, Newman G. The protection of calves against infection with Salmonella Typhimurium by means of a vaccine prepared from Salmonella Dublin (strain 51). Vet Rec 1967;80(25):720–6.
51. Smith BP, Reine-Guerra M, Stocker BA, et al. Vaccination of calves against Salmonella Dublin with aromatic-dependent Salmonella Typhimurium. Am J Vet Res 1984;45(9):1858–61.
52. Jiang Z, De Y, Chang J, et al. Induction of potential protective immunity against enterotoxemia in calves by single or multiple recombinant Clostridium perfringens toxoids. Microbiol Immunol 2014;58(11):621–7.
53. Harris TL, Liang Y, Sharon KP, et al. Influence of Saccharomyces cerevisiae fermentation products, SmartCare in milk replacer and Original XPC in calf starter, on the performance and health of preweaned Holstein calves challenged with Salmonella enterica serotype Typhimurium. J Dairy Sci 2017;100(9):7154–64.
54. Brewer MT, Anderson KL, Yoon I, et al. Amelioration of salmonellosis in preweaned dairy calves fed Saccharomyces cerevisiae fermentation products in feed and milk replacer. Vet Microbiol 2014;172(1–2):248–55.
55. Magalhães VJA, Susca F, Lima FS, et al. Effect of feeding yeast culture on performance, health, and immunocompetence of dairy calves. J Dairy Sci 2008;91(4): 1497–509.
56. von Buenau R, Jaekel L, Schubotz E, et al. Escherichia coli strain Nissle 1917: significant reduction of neonatal calf diarrhea. J Dairy Sci 2005;88(1):317–23.
57. Marcondes MI, Pereira TR, Chagas JCC, et al. Performance and health of Holstein calves fed different levels of milk fortified with symbiotic complex containing pre- and probiotics. Trop Anim Health Prod 2016;48(8):1555–60.

58. Chang MN, Wei JY, Hao LY, et al. Effects of different types of zinc supplement on the growth, incidence of diarrhea, immune function, and rectal microbiota of newborn dairy calves. J Dairy Sci 2020;103(7):6100–13.
59. Feldmann HR, Williams DR, Champagne JD, et al. Effectiveness of zinc supplementation on diarrhea and average daily gain in pre-weaned dairy calves: A double-blind, block-randomized, placebo-controlled clinical trial. PLoS One 2019;14(7):e0219321.
60. Vega CG, Bok M, Ebinger M, et al. A new passive immune strategy based on IgY antibodies as a key element to control neonatal calf diarrhea in dairy farms. BMC Vet Res 2020;16(1):264.

Cryptosporidiosis

Pamela R.F. Adkins, DVM, MS, PhD

KEYWORDS

- Cryptosporidium • Diarrhea • Preweaned calf • Pathophysiology • Management

KEY POINTS

- Cryptosporidiosis, primarily caused by *Cryptosporidium parvum*, is a very common cause of diarrhea in preweaned dairy calves.
- *Cryptosporidium* is spread primarily by fecal-oral transmission and good hygiene is imperative to prevent the spread.
- Oocysts are very hardy in the environment, but they are susceptible to high temperatures and drying.
- Diagnosis can help producers understand important risk factors and prevention steps. Treatment of the individual animal is often nonspecific supportive care.

INTRODUCTION

Gastrointestinal disease in preweaned dairy calves continues to result in economic loss and mortality. Cryptosporidiosis is endemic in cattle worldwide and is globally one of the most common causes of diarrhea in dairy calves during the first 3 weeks of life. It is a zoonotic multifactorial disease, and many risk factors related to the calf, the environment, and production practices are involved.

CRYPTOSPORIDIUM SPECIES IN CALVES

Cryptosporidium is a ubiquitous intestinal protozoan parasite. There are approximately 40 named species of *Cryptosporidium*, with most species having host specificity.[1] Humans are primarily infected with *Cryptosporidium parvum* and *Cryptosporidium hominis*, whereas cattle are infected with *C parvum*, *Cryptosporidium bovis*, *Cryptosporidium ryanae*, and *Cryptosporidium andersoni*. *C andersoni* is more frequently found in adult cattle and infects the abomasum,[2] whereas *C bovis* and *C ryanae* are primarily identified in weaned calves.[3] In most geographic regions that have been evaluated, *C parvum* is the primary species associated with clinical disease in neonatal calves. There are exceptions to this, as some countries, such as Sweden, have reported *C bovis* as the dominant species in preweaned dairy calves.[4] *C*

Department of Veterinary Medicine and Surgery, University of Missouri, 900 E Campus Drive, Columbia, MO 65211, USA
E-mail address: adkinsp@missouri.edu

Vet Clin Food Anim 38 (2022) 121–131
https://doi.org/10.1016/j.cvfa.2021.11.009
0749-0720/22/© 2021 Elsevier Inc. All rights reserved.

parvum is one of the few *Cryptosporidium* species with a broad host range and is the most important zoonotic species.[1]

CRYPTOSPORIDIUM TRANSMISSION AND PATHOGENESIS

In general, cryptosporidiosis is spread by fecal-oral transmission, often involving contaminated water or food supply or via insect vectors.[5,6] Following ingestion of oocysts, the low pH of the gastrointestinal tract and warm body temperature trigger oocysts excystation, and 4 sporozoites are released. The sporozoites adhere to epithelial cells of the ileum and then become incorporated within a parasitophorous vacuole formed by the host cell membrane, remaining extracytoplasmic. Within the vacuole, the parasite is able to obtain necessary nutrients from the host while being protected from the host immune response, as well as the hostile gut environment. The parasite begins asexual and then sexual reproductive cycles, releasing different life stages of the parasite that are able to reinfect the host through invasion of neighboring epithelial cells. Thick-walled oocysts are produced, shed in the feces, and are immediately infective to other hosts.[7]

Cryptosporidium causes diarrhea through parasite invasion and destruction of the small intestinal epithelium, resulting in villus atrophy and crypt hyperplasia that lead to impaired digestion and transport, resulting in malabsorption diarrhea.[8] Lesions are primarily found in the distal small intestines but can also be in the cecum, colon, and duodenum.[9] Animals of all ages can be infected, but diarrhea is mainly associated with preweaned calves. Calves infected with *Cryptosporidium partum* can be asymptomatic or develop severe diarrhea and dehydration. Infected animals generally shed large numbers (1×10^{10}) of infective oocysts in the feces.[10] The infectious dose can be as low as 17 oocysts, with some strain variability.[11] The prevalence of *Cryptosporidium* shedding is high among calves 7 to 21 days old, with the highest prevalence found among calves younger than 2 weeks.[12,13] Calves begin shedding oocysts as early as 2 days of age, with peak shedding occurring at 14 days of age.[5] The onset of diarrhea is generally 3 to 4 days after ingestion of infective oocysts and lasts 1 to 2 weeks.[7] Higher infectious doses are associated with more severe disease and potentially higher losses.[11]

EPIDEMIOLOGY

A large-scale survey that evaluated 2545 preweaned dairy heifer calves from 104 operations in 13 states identified that almost all operations had at least 1 calf positive for *Cryptosporidium* (94.2%). Overall, 43% of calves tested were positive for *Cryptosporidium*.[14] *Cryptosporidium* is more prevalent among young calves, with 63% of calves younger than 2 weeks testing positive and only 9% of calves older than 6 weeks testing positive.[13]

RISK FACTORS
Calf-Level Risk Factors

Calf-specific risk factors that have been considered include breed, sex, birth weight, twinning, whether the dam was multiparous, average daily weight gain, protein intake, fat intake, whether the calf's navel was disinfected, and whether the calves were dehorned.[13,18] Currently there is no clear support for these to be considered significant factors associated with cryptosporidiosis.[13,18] Calves given *Escherichia coli* bacterins, toxoids, or other vaccines designed to prevent calf diarrhea have been found to be at increased risk of cryptosporidiosis (**Table 1**). This is not because these immune

Table 1
Important factors involved in increasing or decreasing the risk of cryptosporidiosis in dairy calves

Factor	Impact	Considerations
Calf level		
Usage of vaccine to help prevent calf diarrhea	Increased risk	Likely because herds with problems use these products[15]
Environment level		
Summer	Increased risk	Increased shedding in feces[13]
Management level		
Large operations	Increased risk	More calves shedding throughout the year[13]
Segregation of cows before calving	Decreased risk	Adult cows can also shed oocysts[16]
Concrete flooring	Decreased risk	Concrete is easier to clean than other flooring types[15]
Soap and water to clean feeding utensils	Decreased risk	Likely related to general cleanliness of farms[15]
Feeding milk replacer	Increased risk	Likely related to fact that large farms often use replacers[15]
Feeding starter grain in first week of life	Increased risk	May be due to sudden start of grain causing disruption in GI microflora[17]

Abbreviation: GI, gastrointestinal.

stimulating products actually cause disease but likely because herds using these products tend to have a history of diarrheal diseases.[15]

Environmental Risk Factors

Season affects the prevalence of *Cryptosporidium*, with an increase in average temperature humidity index being associated with an increase in detection of *Cryptosporidium* in fecal samples (see **Table 1**).[13] In one study, 55% of calves tested positive for *Cryptosporidium* in October and only 36% were positive in March.[13]

In general, the environment is a major factor to consider regarding cryptosporidiosis because the parasite can easily survive through many environmental conditions. *Cryptosporidium* is difficult to remove from the environment, as the oocysts have a tough outer shell, enabling survival against many commonly used farm disinfectants. Oocysts are resistant to chlorination of water and have also been shown to survive in silage.[19] The oocysts can survive for long periods of time in a wide range of temperatures ($-22°C$ to $60°C$).[20,21] At temperatures less than $15°C$ ($59°F$), oocysts can maintain infectivity for as long as a year.[22] Higher temperatures result in more rapid inactivation, within 21 days and 72 hours at $30°C$ ($86°F$) and $37°C$ ($98.6°F$), respectively.[23] Desiccation does prove lethal with most of the oocysts dying after being air-dried for 2 hours at room temperature. Conversely, the oocysts can survive for long periods of time in water, up to 12 weeks at $4°C$ ($39°F$).[24]

Management Risk Factors

Based on a large data set, geographic location of a herd has some impact on the disease, as *Cryptosporidium* positive samples are more commonly detected among calves sampled in the Western United States compared with the Eastern region;

this is likely related to operational size, as most dairy farms in the Western states are considered large. More calves test positive on large operations compared with both medium and small operations (see **Table 1**).[13] It was hypothesized that large operations have more calves shedding the organism because they have a greater number of calves throughout the year and may have more calves shedding at approximately 2 weeks of age, while simultaneously having younger susceptible calves.[13]

Because infection occurs via the fecal-oral route, husbandry practices are related to infection and transmission (see **Table 1**). Numerous management factors have been found to be associated with the risk of *Cryptosporidium parvum* shedding in dairy calves. Segregation of the cow from the rest of the herd before calving can be protective.[16] This is likely related to the fact that adult cows can shed *C parvum*, and carrier cows are likely a source of infection. Reducing the number of cows that calves are exposed to reduces the chance for infection. Concrete flooring for calves reduces the risk, whereas earth or gravel flooring increases the risk of cryptosporidiosis, because concrete is easier to clean.[15] Farms using soap or detergent when washing feeding utensils have a lower prevalence of *C parvum*, related to higher quality hygiene in general. Feeding a starter grain in the first week of life also increases the risk of cryptosporidiosis. This finding has been recognized in several studies and may be due to grain causing a disruption in the gastrointestinal (GI) microflora, which then results in increased shedding of *C parvum*.[15,17] In addition, feeding a milk replacer to calves in the first week of life is associated with an increased prevalence of *C parvum*. This finding may be related to farm size, as larger herds are more likely to use milk replacers.[15]

CLINICAL PRESENTATION

The main clinical presentation of *C parvum* in calves is diarrhea. Other clinical signs can include depression, dehydration, decreased feed intake, abdominal pain, and potentially tenesmus. The severity and duration of disease are highly variable. Several factors are involved regarding severity of clinical disease, including *C parvum* dose, immune status, nutritional status, virulence of the pathogen, and the occurrence of co-infections.[7,11,25] Co-infections with other enteric pathogens have been documented to contribute to the severity of cryptosporidiosis.[26] Calves with severe cases can take 4 to 6 weeks to fully recover; however, mortality is generally low.[14]

DIAGNOSIS

A diagnosis of *Cryptosporidium* can be made through detection of the oocysts through microscopic examination, the *C parvum* antigen using immunoassays, or *Cryptosporidium* DNA in the feces using polymerase chain reaction testing (PCR). In general, the oocysts are stable in feces for several days at room temperature, allowing identification of the parasite within samples that need to be shipped to a diagnostic laboratory. Microscopy is the most commonly used method of detecting active infections and is the only technique that can distinguish the presence of oocysts. Although this is a cost-effective method of diagnosis, accuracy can be affected by fecal consistency, slide preparation, and interpretation.[27] *Cryptosporidium* oocysts are small (4–6 um in diameter) and can be easily missed. Furthermore, microscopy methods do not provide speciation of the parasite. Advanced preparation and staining techniques have been developed to improve detection. Fecal floatation with Sheather's sugar solution is the most sensitive and specific preparation technique, allowing concentration of the protozoa.[28] Modified acid-fast stains help detect oocysts. Acid-fast staining options that are often used include the Ziehl-Neelsen stain or the modified Kinyoun stain

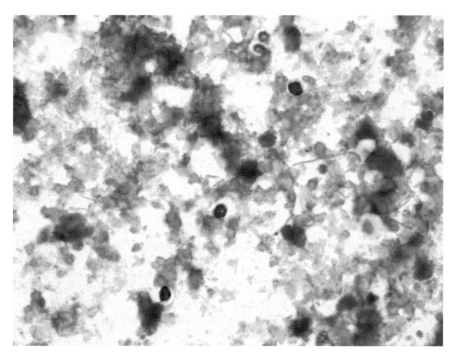

Fig. 1. *Cryptosporidium* from a fecal smear stained with modified Kinyoun acid fast stain. This preparation was made without fecal flotation. (*Courtesy of* Dr Angela Royal, University of Missouri Veterinary Clinical Pathology Service.)

(**Fig. 1**). Usage of a safranin methylene blue staining has been shown to help better differentiate oocysts and yeast.[28]

Many immunoassays have been developed to detect *Cryptosporidium*. Enzyme immunoassays require reduced labor, time, and microscopic skills; however, the sensitivity and specificity vary. One study evaluated the diagnostic sensitivity and specificity of different assays and found that immunofluorescence microscopy was significantly more sensitive than other methods. Immunofluorescence microscopy is significantly more expensive than other microscopy-based methods and requires a fluorescence microscope.[29] Several dipstick immunoassays have also been developed, and although they have lower sensitivity, they provide a practical alternative to laboratory diagnosis of cryptosporidiosis.[30]

Molecular tools are most frequently used in research settings. They will likely become more common in diagnostic settings. Traditional PCR methods only report the presence or absence of *Cryptosporidium* species, but they can identify the infecting species; these are useful data, as each species has different epidemiology, risk factors, and clinical manifestations. If only traditional PCR that identify *C parvum* are used, mixed infections could go undetected. Speciation of *Cryptosporidium* can be done using multiplex PCR, which could identify mixed infections. Other methods of speciation include enzyme digestion of PCR products (PCR-restriction fragment length polymorphism) or sequencing of gene fragments. Quantitative PCR (qPCR) can also be used to quantify parasite burden.[31] Multiplex qPCR has also been developed to allow the detection of all major enteric pathogens at one time, allowing quantification as well as identification of mixed infections.[32]

TREATMENT

Calf diarrhea is most often treated as undifferentiated, as treatment strategies are similar among the pathogens. Cryptosporidiosis is normally self-limiting in neonatal calves but often requires supportive care such as replacement of lost fluids and electrolytes, reestablishment of acid-base balance, and antiinflammatories. Specific treatment recommendations for undifferentiated calf diarrhea are well described elsewhere.[33,34] Specific therapies for *Cryptosporidium* are activities being researched and may prove beneficial in some cases.

Specific Therapies

Halofuginone lactate, a coccidiostat that functions as a synthetic enzyme inhibitor, has been evaluated as a treatment of *Cryptosporidium* and is labeled for the treatment of cryptosporidiosis in Canada and Europe. This medication is not labeled for use in the United States. A recent systematic review and meta-analysis was conducted to review the efficacy of halofuginone products to treat and prevent cryptosporidiosis in calves.[35] The systematic review showed that prophylactic use of halofuginone products reduces oocysts shedding, diarrhea, and calf mortality. The prophylactic use of this product on farms with confirmed cryptosporidiosis in calves between 12 and 48 hours old can reduce morbidity and mortality.[35] One limitation of this therapy is that it cannot be given to calves that are weak, dehydrated, or have had diarrhea for more than 24 hours[36]; this limits the suitability of this medication to be used for therapeutic purposes. If a producer determines that cryptosporidiosis is a component of the diarrhea problem within their herd, this medication may provide benefits for those calves that have not yet shown clinical symptoms.[35] A second limitation of this product is its toxicity: it is toxic at twice the recommended dose. Symptoms of toxicity include diarrhea, blood in the feces, decline in milk consumption, dehydration, and weakness.[36] These clinical signs may be difficult to differentiate from disease associated with primary enteric pathogens. Using the recommended dosage and determining an accurate weight of the treated animal are important steps before administration. This product can also cause skin allergies for people who handle it and can be dangerous to fish or other aquatic organisms. Usage of gloves when administering the medication and appropriate disposal of unused product or waste are essential.[36] Although this product reduces oocyst shedding, it does not completely prevent it, suggesting that additional hygiene measures are still needed to help control transmission.

A second medication that has shown promise is azithromycin, a macrolide antimicrobial. Azithromycin effectively reduces oocysts shedding and improves clinical signs and weight gain.[37] This antibiotic is used widely in the United States for treatment of respiratory disease in humans, and alternative nonantimicrobial therapies should be considered first. In addition, this medication is relatively expensive. Currently, there are no licensed drugs in the United States to treat cryptosporidiosis. Supportive care is currently the mainstay of treatment.

LONG-TERM IMPACTS

The 120-day risk of mortality following diagnosis of diarrhea in dairy calves is approximately 11% and generally not associated with a specific pathogen (exception: *Salmonella* has a higher mortality risk).[26] Although mortality is generally relatively low, severe clinical cryptosporidiosis at a young age significantly reduces the long-term growth rate of calves.[38,39] Weight lost during the acute infection in neonatal calves is not regained during the subsequent 6 months, indicating a significant economic impact.[39]

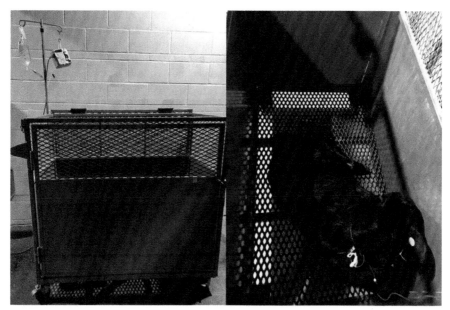

Fig. 2. Picture of a calf being treated for undifferentiated calf diarrhea in isolation. The isolated crate is metal and on concrete to allow for easy disinfection.

Management regimens to reduce the prevalence of this disease among calves will prove beneficial to the producer.

PREVENTION AND CONTROL

The environmental stability of the organism, low infective dose, and high level of excreted oocysts among infected calves make cryptosporidiosis very difficult to control. Measures to try to reduce environmental contamination may include isolation of sick calves, by usage of crates with slatted flooring over concrete, as both surfaces can easily be disinfected (**Fig. 2**). Other important steps include frequent removal of fecal material and contaminated bedding; steam cleaning; and usage of an appropriate disinfectant to clean hutches, crates, and tools. These procedures will reduce environmental buildup of infective oocysts. Disinfectants that may prove useful include 6% or 7.5% hydrogen peroxide at a contact time of 20 minutes.[40] The oocysts are susceptible to heat shock or desiccation. Thoroughly cleaning with very hot water and allowing complete drying can be an effective way to clean materials.

Neutralizing antibodies in colostrum and milk have the potential to reduce infectivity by immobilization of the parasite, blockage of invasion, inhibition of adhesion to host cells, or direct cytotoxicity to *Cryptosporidium* sporozoites.[41] Evidence is limited that colostrum can ever contain enough antibodies to be effective in this manner.[42] In general, there is weak evidence that colostrum ingestion is protective against *C parvum* infection, and there is no consistent evidence that any specific feed delivery system is riskier or more protective.[18] That said, in general, although colostrum may not specifically protect against *Cryptosporidium*, serum immunoglobulin G (IgG) levels and passive transfer of immunity are directly associated with morbidity and mortality. As serum IgG concentrations increase, the likelihood of disease and death decreases.[43] Calves with a serum IgG concentration less than 10 g/L (equivalent of a total protein of

< 5.1 g/dL) are considered to have failure of passive transfer and are at increased risk of disease and death. Serum IgG concentration has a dose-dependent effect, and targeting an IgG concentration of 25 g/L (equivalent of a total protein of $\geq$ 6.2 g/dL) may reduce overall morbidity and mortality in dairy calves.[44]

One research trial compared 2 oz. (56.7 g) daily intake of either bovine serum or soy protein concentrate fed in addition to a whey-based milk replacers to calves orally inoculated with C parvum oocysts. Supplementation of serum reduced oocysts shed and peak scour volume, and a chromium-ethylenediaminetetraacetic acid assay method also indicated a reduction in gut permeability with serum supplementation. Calves were sacrificed at day 18, and it was determined that supplementation of serum improved crypt depth and villous surface area.[45]

ZOONOTIC RISK

People working with diarrheic calves should be warned of the risk of zoonotic disease. Outbreaks of cryptosporidiosis have been described among previously healthy people working in veterinary medical teaching hospitals after admission of calves from farms that were experiencing neonatal diarrhea. In one report, most people who became ill were in direct contact with the diarrheic calves; however, one person became infected after handling soiled clothing.[46] An additional risk for veterinary students has been linked to fetotomy exercises, especially when using dead calves with high fecal Cryptosporidium loads. These studies highlight the importance of personal protective equipment (PPE) and appropriate hand washing with soap and water.[47]

CLINICS CARE POINTS

- Diagnosis is often made using microscopic evaluation of fecal samples, often done in a diagnostic laboratory. Dipstick immunoassays have lower sensitivity but can be easily used by practicing veterinarians.
- Diagnosis of cryptosporidiosis can help the veterinarian guide the producer regarding ways to reduce the transmission of the organism within their herd based on well-established risk factors.
- Using appropriate PPE is important during treatment of these cases, as it is a zoonotic disease.

DISCLOSURE

The author declares that they have no relevant or material financial interest and received no funding in relation to this work.

REFERENCES

1. Feng Y, Ryan UM, Xiao L. Genetic diversity and population structure of cryptosporidium. Trends Parasitol 2018;34:997–1011.
2. Lindsay DS, Upton SJ, Owens DS, et al. Cryptosporidium andersoni n. sp. (Apicomplexa: Cryptosporiidae) from cattle, Bos taurus. J Eukaryot Microbiol 2000; 47:91–5.
3. Santin M, Trout JM, Xiao L, et al. Prevalence and age-related variation of Cryptosporidium species and genotypes in dairy calves. Vet Parasitol 2004;122:103–17.

4. Silverlas C, Bosaeus-Reineck H, Naslund K, et al. Is there a need for improved Cryptosporidium diagnostics in Swedish calves? Int J Parasitol 2013;43:155–61.
5. Olson ME, O'Handley RM, Ralston BJ, et al. Update on Cryptosporidium and Giardia infections in cattle. Trends Parasitol 2004;20:185–91.
6. Graczyk TK, Grimes BH, Knight R, et al. Detection of Cryptosporidium parvum and Giardia lamblia carried by synanthropic flies by combined fluorescent in situ hybridization and a monoclonal antibody. Am J Trop Med Hyg 2003;68: 228–32.
7. Thomson S, Hamilton CA, Hope JC, et al. Bovine cryptosporidiosis: impact, host-parasite interaction and control strategies. Vet Res 2017;48:42.
8. Di Genova BM, Tonelli RR. Infection Strategies of Intestinal Parasite Pathogens and Host Cell Responses. Front Microbiol 2016;7:256.
9. Sanford SE, Josephson GK. Bovine Cryptosporidiosis: Clinical and Pathological Findings in Forty-two Scouring Neonatal Calves. Can Vet J 1982;23:343–7.
10. Nydam DV, Wade SE, Schaaf SL, et al. Number of Cryptosporidium parvum oo-cysts or Giardia spp cysts shed by dairy calves after natural infection. Am J Vet Res 2001;62:1612–5.
11. Zambriski JA, Nydam DV, Wilcox ZJ, et al. Cryptosporidium parvum: determination of ID(5)(0) and the dose-response relationship in experimentally challenged dairy calves. Vet Parasitol 2013;197:104–12.
12. de Graaf DC, Vanopdenbosch E, Ortega-Mora LM, et al. A review of the importance of cryptosporidiosis in farm animals. Int J Parasitol 1999;29:1269–87.
13. Urie NJ, Lombard JE, Shivley CB, et al. Preweaned heifer management on US dairy operations: Part III. Factors associated with Cryptosporidium and Giardia in preweaned dairy heifer calves. J Dairy Sci 2018;101:9199–213.
14. Urie NJ, Lombard JE, Shivley CB, et al. Preweaned heifer management on US dairy operations: Part I. Descriptive characteristics of preweaned heifer raising practices. J Dairy Sci 2018;101:9168–84.
15. Trotz-Williams LA, Martin SW, Leslie KE, et al. Association between management practices and within-herd prevalence of Cryptosporidium parvum shedding on dairy farms in southern Ontario. Prev Vet Med 2008;83:11–23.
16. Silverlas C, Emanuelson U, de Verdier K, et al. Prevalence and associated management factors of Cryptosporidium shedding in 50 Swedish dairy herds. Prev Vet Med 2009;90:242–53.
17. Maldonado-Camargo S, Atwill ER, Saltijeral-Oaxaca JA, et al. Prevalence of and risk factors for shedding of Cryptosporidium parvum in Holstein Freisian dairy calves in central Mexico. Prev Vet Med 1998;36:95–107.
18. Brainard J, Hooper L, McFarlane S, et al. Systematic review of modifiable risk factors shows little evidential support for most current practices in Cryptosporidium management in bovine calves. Parasitol Res 2020;119:3571–84.
19. Merry RJ, Mawdsley JL, Brooks AE, et al. Viability of Cryptosporidium parvum during ensilage of perennial ryegrass. J Appl Microbiol 1997;82:115–20.
20. Fujino T, Matsui T, Kobayashi F, et al. The effect of heating against Cryptosporidium oocysts. J Vet Med Sci 2002;64:199–200.
21. Casemore DP. Epidemiological aspects of human cryptosporidiosis. Epidemiol Infect 1990;104:1–28.
22. King BJ, Monis PT. Critical processes affecting Cryptosporidium oocyst survival in the environment. Parasitology 2007;134:309–23.
23. King BJ, Keegan AR, Monis PT, et al. Environmental temperature controls Cryptosporidium oocyst metabolic rate and associated retention of infectivity. Appl Environ Microbiol 2005;71:3848–57.

24. Robertson LJ, Campbell AT, Smith HV. Survival of Cryptosporidium parvum oocysts under various environmental pressures. Appl Environ Microbiol 1992;58: 3494–500.

25. Meganck V, Hoflack G, Opsomer G. Advances in prevention and therapy of neonatal dairy calf diarrhoea: a systematical review with emphasis on colostrum management and fluid therapy. Acta Vet Scand 2014;56:75.

26. Barkley JA, Pempek JA, Bowman AS, et al. Longitudinal health outcomes for enteric pathogens in preweaned calves on Ohio dairy farms. Prev Vet Med 2021;190:105323.

27. Keserue HA, Fuchslin HP, Wittwer M, et al. Comparison of rapid methods for detection of Giardia spp. and Cryptosporidium spp. (oo)cysts using transportable instrumentation in a field deployment. Environ Sci Technol 2012;46:8952–9.

28. Rekha KM, Puttalakshmamma GC, D'Souza PE. Comparison of different diagnostic techniques for the detection of cryptosporidiosis in bovines. Vet World 2016;9:211–5.

29. Chalmers RM, Campbell BM, Crouch N, et al. Comparison of diagnostic sensitivity and specificity of seven cryptosporidium assays used in the UK. J Med Microbiol 2011;60:1598–604.

30. Geurden T, Claerebout E, Vercruysse J, et al. A Bayesian evaluation of four immunological assays for the diagnosis of clinical cryptosporidiosis in calves. Vet J 2008;176:400–2.

31. Hadfield SJ, Robinson G, Elwin K, et al. Detection and differentiation of Cryptosporidium spp. in human clinical samples by use of real-time PCR. J Clin Microbiol 2011;49:918–24.

32. Cho YI, Kim WI, Liu S, et al. Development of a panel of multiplex real-time polymerase chain reaction assays for simultaneous detection of major agents causing calf diarrhea in feces. J Vet Diagn Invest 2010;22:509–17.

33. Constable PD. Treatment of calf diarrhea: antimicrobial and ancillary treatments. Vet Clin North Am Food Anim Pract 2009;25:101–20, vi.

34. Smith GW, Berchtold J. Fluid therapy in calves. Vet Clin North Am Food Anim Pract 2014;30:409–27, vi.

35. Brainard J, Hammer CC, Hunter PR, et al. Efficacy of halofuginone products to prevent or treat cryptosporidiosis in bovine calves: a systematic review and meta-analyses. Parasitology 2021;148:408–19.

36. European Medicines Agency. Halocur. Available: https://www.ema.europa.eu/en/medicines/veterinary/EPAR/halocur Visited. May 19, 2021.

37. Elitok B, Elitok OM, Pulat H. Efficacy of azithromycin dihydrate in treatment of cryptosporidiosis in naturally infected dairy calves. J Vet Intern Med 2005;19: 590–3.

38. Pardon B, Hostens M, Duchateau L, et al. Impact of respiratory disease, diarrhea, otitis and arthritis on mortality and carcass traits in white veal calves. BMC Vet Res 2013;9:79.

39. Shaw HJ, Innes EA, Morrison LJ, et al. Long-term production effects of clinical cryptosporidiosis in neonatal calves. Int J Parasitol 2020;50:371–6.

40. Barbee SL, Weber DJ, Sobsey MD, et al. Inactivation of Cryptosporidium parvum oocyst infectivity by disinfection and sterilization processes. Gastrointest Endosc 1999;49:605–11.

41. Jenkins MC. Advances and prospects for subunit vaccines against protozoa of veterinary importance. Vet Parasitol 2001;101:291–310.

42. Burton AJ, Nydam DV, Jones G, et al. Antibody responses following administration of a Cryptosporidium parvum rCP15/60 vaccine to pregnant cattle. Vet Parasitol 2011;175:178–81.
43. Urie NJ, Lombard JE, Shivley CB, et al. Preweaned heifer management on US dairy operations: Part V. Factors associated with morbidity and mortality in preweaned dairy heifer calves. J Dairy Sci 2018;101:9229–44.
44. Lombard J, Urie N, Garry F, et al. Consensus recommendations on calf- and herd-level passive immunity in dairy calves in the United States. J Dairy Sci 2020;103:7611–24.
45. Hunt E, Qiang F, Armstrong M, et al. Oral bovine serum concentrate improves cryptosporidial enteritis in calves. Pediatr Res 2002;51:370–6.
46. Reif JS, Wimmer L, Smith JA, et al. Human cryptosporidiosis associated with an epizootic in calves. Am J Public Health 1989;79:1528–30.
47. Thomas-Lopez D, Muller L, Vestergaard LS, et al. Veterinary Students Have a Higher Risk of Contracting Cryptosporidiosis when Calves with High Fecal Cryptosporidium Loads Are Used for Fetotomy Exercises. Appl Environ Microbiol 2020;86.

Milk Replacer Ingredients
What and Why?

Dave Wood, MBA

KEYWORDS

- Milk replacer ingredients • Dairy calf nutrition • Calf milk replacer • Whole milk

KEY POINTS

- The protein, carbohydrate, fatty acid, vitamin, and mineral requirements of the preruminant calf should be met using highly digestible, wholesome, water-dispersible calf milk replacer (CMR) ingredients that optimize health and growth.
- Protein represents the largest ingredient expense in a CMR (typically 70%) and special care should be taken to use proven, consistent, suitable sources.
- Lactose should provide all or nearly all carbohydrates in a CMR formula. Fresh, edible-grade fats and oils in sources that will not separate in milk and that mimic the fatty acid profile of butter should be used.
- Clean, wholesome whole milk, although a near-perfect food for the calf, is inadequate in vitamin and trace mineral nutrition.
- Extending the feeding of colostrum and transition milk is shown to improve gut health and reduce diarrhea. The addition of spray-dried bovine plasma is shown to cost-effectively mimic this practice.
- Practitioners should advise clients to purchase from reputable milk replacer manufacturers who consistently formulate using ingredients suitable for the milk-fed calf.

 Video content accompanies this article at http://www.vetfood.theclinics.com.

INTRODUCTION

The CMR industry was established post-World War II in both Europe and in North America. The establishment of the special milk-fed veal industry in the 1970s and 80s paved the way for improvements in milk replacer ingredients, manufacturing know-how, and milk replacer feeding practices. The nonveal milk replacer market

Statistical testing in trials referenced in this article was not always similar. The author of this article has listed those values in the text considered important to the interpretation of outcomes, with trends being $P \leq .10$, significant being $P \leq .05$, and highly significant declared at $P \leq .01$. The significance values are reported as presented in the papers reviewed.
Director of Sales and Technical Support, Animix, Juneau, Wisconsin 172 Cross Street, Juneau, WI, USA
E-mail address: biowood10@gmail.com

has expanded over the past decade. This occurred at least partially because increased prewean body weight gains are associated with increased future milk production. Pressure to achieve consistent high health status and enhanced early growth has resulted in further need to assure CMR ingredient quality and consistency.

The calf is the dairy's future. Also, there is heightened consumer and regulatory pressure to eliminate the practice of feeding antibiotic-contaminated waste milk. In the future, the need for bovine practitioners to advise clients on their milk replacer selection, and milk feeding strategies will become even more important.

The goal of this article is to provide practical science-based advice on suitable components of a consistent, quality performance-oriented milk replacer.

GENERAL GUIDELINES

Milk replacer ingredients are commonly derived from whey. Ingredients used in milk replacers should be derived from fresh product streams that have not had an opportunity to spoil or denature before preservation via spray drying. Ingredients should be low in standard plate count and void of mold and pathogens. Scorched particles and denatured proteins should be avoided. Ingredients should disperse adequately for the specific milk mix system used on a farm. Ingredients should not float, stick to mixing, and feeding equipment or settle out within reasonable milk feeding periods.

Specific guidelines for each nutrient category are outlined later in discussion.

PROTEIN – CLINIC CARE POINTS

- High-quality milk (casein- or whey-based) and plasma proteins are proven to perform during all stages of milk feeding. Both are widely used in N. American milk replacer formulas.
- Transition milk is biologically normal. Disease challenge trials (*Cryptosporidium parvum,* bovine coronavirus, and *E coli)* demonstrate improved health and performance of calves when immunoglobulin-dense plasma protein-based products are added to CMR.
- Hydrolyzed wheat gluten protein when used to replace 15% to 20% of the milk protein in the CMR formula can perform comparably to an all-milk protein formula, however, results (particularly in the first weeks of life) are not consistent as several trials demonstrate relatively poorer performance.[1]
- Use of inadequately processed soy results in intestinal damage, reduced enzyme production, relatively poorer digestibility, and reduced daily gain when used in CMR's. Antigenic proteins are absorbed, and such products are not suitable for use.[1] Soy products must be assured void of β conglycinin, be extremely low in antitryptic activity and have low polysaccharide content.[1]

CASEIN OR WHEY?

A common milk protein source used in modern milk replacer formulas is whey protein concentrate (WPC). WPC is typically commercially available as 34% crude protein (**Table 1**). High protein WPC (commonly 80% CP) is also suitable for use. Significant protein contribution also comes from sweet whey which is typically 12% CP (see **Table 1**).

Skim milk powder (a.k.a. dried skim milk), although highly suitable for use in CMR is typically more expensive compared with WPC. Typically, skim milk protein is 34% CP (see **Table 1**).

Table 1
Typical specifications of suitable milk replacer protein, fat, and lactose sources

Ingredient & Source	Crude protein (%)	Crude fat (%)	Fiber (%)	Ash (%)	Lactose (%)	Dry Matter (%)
Whey protein concentrate 34%, Milk Specialties Global	34%	3%	0%	5.95%	52.10%	not listed
Skimmed milk powder, Melkweg, VanDrie, NL	34%	0.7%	0%	8.2%	51%	96%
Sweet whey powder spray-dried Melkweg, VanDrie, NL	11.0-<13.0%	1.5%	0%	8 - <9.5%	68 - <75%	96%
7/60 HI-FAT, Milk Specialties Global	7%	60%	0%	4%	not listed	98%
NutraPro-UV Bovine Plasma, APC	min. 78%	0.30%	max. 0.5%	max 10%	0%	92%
ADM Nutrior 201 wheat protein	≥81.0%	2%–4%	0.4%–0.8%	≤1.5%	0%	≥95%
ADM Soycomil K (2 ppm β-conElycinin)	65%	1%	3.5%	6.5%	0%	91% min.

In the 1980s, the merits of WPC- and skim milk-based formulas were heatedly debated, and this debate continues to a lesser degree today; however, digestibility studies in calves show that both perform well and comparably (**Table 2**).

TRANSITION MILK

Assisting dairies with colostrum management is arguably one of the best ways a practitioner can improve calf health and growth on-farm and encouraging the supplementation of antibodies in milk or milk replacer is an additional way to extend this endeavor.

Research shows a significant quantity of circulating antibodies go into the gastrointestinal tract of the calf daily. The transfer to the gastrointestinal tract of circulating (serum) IgG antibodies labeled with ^{125}I was monitored in newborn calves and determined to be approximately 4% daily,[10] meaning a calf with a reserve of 100 g of circulatory IgG from maternal colostrum excretes 4 g of immunoglobulins (IgG) daily into its digestive tract.

In nature, and before the consolidation of the dairy industry, calves were commonly fed transition milk (a blend of milk and colostrum) for several days before transitioning to a diet composed solely of whole milk and reestablishing this practice via feeding IgG-dense proteins has become popular.

Table 2
Milk-fed calf protein digestibility research examples

Protein source	n	CP%	CMR intake g/d	Age of calves (d)	%of CP.	CP Digestibility (%)	Citation
Skim milk	5	26.5%	app. 700	3–8	100%	87.0%	Grongnet et al,[2] 1981 (INRA, France, veal)
WPC (balance skim milk)	5	26.2%	app. 700	3–8	57.3%	85.9%	[2]
WPC, further heat-treated (balance skim milk)	5	26.2%	app. 700	3–8	57.3%	88.8%	
Skim milk	5	26.5%	app. 1000	28–33	100%	97.0%	
WPC (balance skim milk)	5	26.2%	app. 1000	28–33	57.3%	92.3%	
WPC, further heat-treated (balance skim milk)	5	26.2%	app. 1000	28–33	57.3%	95.0%	
WPC	10	22.5%	app. 875	21–28	100%	82.2%	Dawson et al,[3] 1988 (Kansas State U)
WPC	10	22.5%	app. 1120	42–49	-	87.5%	[3]
Skim milk	5	-	-	8–14	-	94.0%	Sturdsholm et al,[6] 1988 (Denmark)
Skim milk with pancreatin stop clotting	5	-	-	8–14	-	90.0%	[6]
Whey powder	5	-	-	8–14	-	87.0%	
Skim milk	7	20.7%	1090	39–44	100%	93.2%	Lalles et al,[4] 1995 (INRA, France, veal)
Skim milk	7	20.7%	2700	95–100	100%	94.4%	[4]
Soy protein isolate	7	20.4%	1090	39–44	72%	89.1%	
Soy protein isolate	7	20.4%	2700	95–100	72%	91.5%	
Heated soy flour	7	20.6%	1090	39–44	72%	67.8%	
Heated soy flour	7	20.6%	2700	95–100	72%	68.6%	
Skim milk	2	21.9%	est. 1700	63–70	100%	92.0%	Toullec et al,[9] 1998 (INRA, France, veal)

Solubilized wheat gluten protein	2	21.8%	est. 1700	63–70	76.3%	85.0%	[9]
Solubilized wheat gluten protein	2	21.9%	est. 1700	63–70	36.2%	89.0%	
Skim milk	4	20.6%	610	Wk 2, 4,8	100%	85.5%	Terosky et al,[7] 1997 (Penn State U) [7]
Skim milk (67%), WPC (33%)	4	21.1%	615	Wk 2, 4,8	mix	87.7%	
WPC (67%), Skim milk (33%)	4	21.1%	632	Wk 2, 4,8	mix	87.9%	
WPC	4	20.7%	609	Wk 2, 4,8	100%	87.9%	
Skim milk (primarily, some whey)	5	22.5%	not reported	35–41	100%	94.1%	Tolman et al,[8] 1991 (ILOB, NL, veal) [8]
Solubilized wheat gluten protein	5	28.0%	not reported	35–41	28.5%	95.3%	
Solubilized wheat gluten protein	5	33.8%	not reported	35–41	47.3%	94.9%	
Milk protein (unsure if WPC or skim)	6	21.8%	11.6 g/kg BW	2–4	-	78.7%	Liang et al,[5] 2016 (Texas Tech, Jerseys) [5]
Milk protein (unsure if WPC or skim)	6	30.8%	19.2 g/kg BW	2–4	-	88.0%	
Milk protein (unsure if WPC or skim)	6	21.8%	11.6 g/kg BW	5–7	-	85.0%	
Milk protein (unsure if WPC or skim)	6	30.8	19.2 g/kg BW	5–7	-	85.3%	

Feeding colostrum post-gut-closure for either 3[11] or 7[12] days postnatal has been shown to increase ($P < .05$) the rate of development of the small intestine. It has also been shown to reduce diarrhea (relative risk = 0.61) and antimicrobial treatments ($P = .02$) and improve ADG ($P = .04$) when fed at 70 g/d (10 g IgG) for 14 days.[13]

Similar effects have been noted in 4 published disease challenge studies when plasma-based IgG-dense proteins were fed to calves. A 75 g/d dose of spray-dried bovine plasma (SDBP) prevented clinical signs of disease when calves were challenged with orally administered virulent strains of E coli.[14] Calves fed sterilized whole milk with no added plasma (control) noted severe diarrhea, fever, loss of appetite, and 100% mortality ($P = .0399$).[14] Calves fed 30 g/d of SDBP noted intermediary morbidity and mortality results.[14]

Compared with calves fed the nonmedicated all-milk protein CMR (negative control), a relatively low 3.3% inclusion of SDBP resulted in an improvement in attitude score ($P = .02$), hydration score ($P = .004$), and in 21 d body weight gain ($P = .02$) when 3 d old calves were orally challenged with enterotoxigenic Escherichia coli.[15] The health-improvement response from supplementing plasma paralleled calves fed CMR with 800:400 g per ton of neomycin/oxytetracycline.[15]

Spray-dried bovine serum is plasma minus fibrinogen, and its addition at a relatively high dose (product contained 32 g bovine serum-based IgG) administered in the CMR at 24-h postoral infection of a virulent coronavirus isolate noted increased packed cell volume ($P < .01$) and a 29.5% improvement in feed intake ($P = .02$).[16] Also, when orally challenged with C parvum at 8 d of age calves supplemented with 57 g/d of spray-dried bovine serum noted a 33% reduction ($P \leq .05$) in diarrhea volume and a nearly 4-fold reduction in oocyst shedding ($P = .03$) at peak illness (d 4–6 postinoculation) than calves supplemented with a comparable protein supplementation from soy isolate.[17] These researchers also noted a 30% reduction in gut permeability ($P \leq .001$) as measured by a chromium EDTA assay and permeability on-par with the unchallenged control group.[17] All calves were killed at 9-days postinfection and calves supplemented bovine serum noted a 15% improvement in both villus surface area ($P = .05$) and crypt depth ($P = .05$) as compared with their soy-fed peers.[17]

Spray-dried bovine plasma (SDBP) is a significant source of antibodies. Animix QA/QC used radial immunodiffusion technique analysis on 568 production lots of APC Nutrapro SDBP and found an average concentration of 22.2 g IgG/100 g of powder (±2.75 SD, results available on request). Postgut-closure, IgG's fed in the milk or CMR are not absorbed, rather, in human patients they have been recovered and shown to be biologically functional at a rate of 19% (±3%) after passage through the gastrointestinal tract.[18]

Videos 1 and 2 provide further information pertaining to the effects of using spray-dried bovine plasma to supplement either whole milk or as a protein source in milk replacer formulas. **Fig. 1** shows the physical appearance of APC Nutrapro B spray-dried bovine plasma powder.

PLANT-BASED PROTEINS

For several decades now, plant-based proteins, primarily hydrolyzed wheat protein, but also, suitable soy, have been extensively used in the milk replacer and veal industry in Europe. This is impressive, as the veal industry in Europe represents more than 5 million calves reared annually.[19] However, a key difference between the EU and in North America is that calves are commonly reared, by law, on the farm of birth for several weeks before being transported to veal farms and are thus likely fed maternal colostrum and whole milk.

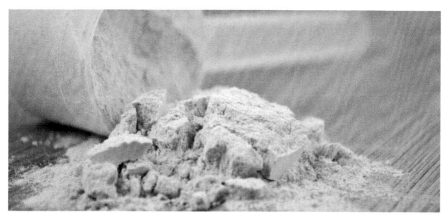

Fig. 1. Spray-dried bovine plasma (NutraPro B, APC). (*From* Animix, Juneau, WI; with permission.)

North Americans can capture the cost-saving strategies of suitable plant-based proteins if used strategically and conservatively. Select sources of hydrolyzed wheat gluten protein are proven highly digestible (see **Table 2**), and wheat is an appealing plant-based alternative because, unlike soy, it is naturally void of antinutritional factors. Care must be taken to supplement appropriate levels of synthetic L-lysine as wheat protein is relatively deficient in this amino acid and, typically, this enhances the savings from the use of wheat.

Recent research examining formulas composed of 6.1% hydrolyzed wheat protein combined with 6.33% spray-dried bovine plasma noted similar performance to an all-milk control.[20] However, some research has noted lesser performance from feeding wheat alone (6% of the formula) or in combination with plasma (3% of each).[21] This is perhaps indicative of the greater variability in performance, particularly in the first weeks of life, associated with the use of plant-based proteins.

Video 3 provides further information regarding the proper utilization of hydrolyzed wheat gluten protein in milk replacer formulas.

The antinutritional factors naturally found in soy such as β conglycinin, must be consistently negated before soy can be a suitable source of protein for use in CMR. The research shown in **Table 3** (From Alternative ingredients in calf milk replacer – a review for bovine practitioners. Bov Pract 2016; 50:65–88; with permission) demonstrates the deleterious effect antinutritional factors in soy can have on protein digestibility.[1].

Improperly processed soy not only hurts protein digestibility, but it also damages gut tissues.[23] When antinutritional factors are nearly void, soy can perform comparably to milk protein.[24]

FURTHER RESOURCES ON SUITABLE PROTEINS FOR USE IN CALF MILK REPLACERS

A review of milk-fed calf research examining the use of spray-dried animal plasma, hydrolyzed wheat, and soy proteins in CMR, encompassing 20, 17, and 26 studies, respectively, was published in *Bovine Practitioner* in 2016[1] and is available at a link in the citation. Also, as formerly mentioned, several videos on the research behind and use of plasma and wheat proteins in CMR's were created by the author (Videos 1–3).

Table 3
Analytical criteria correlated with reduction in apparent digestibility of soy protein in preruminant calves[22]

Commercial Soy Product (Lalles et al, 1996. JDS 79:475)	Digestibility (%)	β-conglycinin (mg/g of CP)***	∝-conglycinin (mg/g of CP)*	Antitrypsin (TUI³/mg CP)*	Native Protein (% of total N)**	Glycinin (mg/g of CP)**
Raw soy flour		155.0	31.5	140.0		269.0
Toasted soy flour 52.9% CP	59	36.1	15.2	19.9	50.9	39.4
Toasted soy flour 52.8% CP	66	13.4	0.45	5.7	17.2	26.8
Toasted soy flour 56.3% CP	76	-	1.13	6.6	15.5	0.7
Water extracted toasted SPC	61	25.5	2.93	6.5	21.6	20.4
Water extracted toasted SPC	71	14.7	3.2	5.2	33.7	32.9
Water extracted toasted SPC	81	-	0.7	2.7	7.9	0.0
Alcohol-extracted heated SPC	81	-	0.45	3.4	9.4	-
Water extracted proteolyzed SPC	82	-	0	2.5	2.9	-
Water extracted proteolyzed SPC	84	-	0.4	1.4	4.4	10.5

Simple linear regression between analytical criteria and apparent digestibility of soybean Nitrogen

*$P < .05$, **$P < .01$, ***$P < .0001$

Analysis of results of four separate trials in calves 2–4 mo of age

n = 5–7 calves per treatment group

CARBOHYDRATES AND LIPIDS – CLINIC CARE POINTS

- Lactose from milk or milk ingredients should provide most or all carbohydrates in the liquid diet.
- Fresh, edible-grade, lard, tallow, palm, and coconut oil should be formulated into a finished fat blend providing a similar fatty acid profile to butterfat.
- Fat should not separate or cream when exposed to routine milk blending or a normal length of time to feed.
- Medium-chain fatty acids in coconut oil are shown to improve digestibility.
- Hydrophilic emulsifiers are used in formulas to stabilize free fat and to improve fat digestibility.

The small intestine of the neonatal calf contains significant quantities of the enzyme lactase and CMR should provide lactose.[25] Sucrase is not present. [25,26] Nonlactose sugars should be minimized in milk replacer formulas.

Fat is a critical energy source for the young calf, in fact, a common inclusion of 20% in milk replacer provides 60% of the digestible energy.[28] It is critical that a suitable replacement for butterfat be used.

Tallow, lard, palm, and coconut oil are shown to be highly digestible in calf milk replacers when appropriate sources and formulations are used (**Table 4**).

Fatty acid profile should mimic butter using economical and suitable fats and oils. **Table 5** compares the fatty acid content of common fats and oils to butter and, also to a typical veal feed fat formula composed of 36% tallow, 36% lard, 20% coconut oil, 6% lecithin, and 2% hydrophilic emulsifier. Note that lard, tallow, or palm oil provide palmitic, stearic, and oleic acids found in butter, while either coconut or palm kernel oil provide caprylic, capric, lauric, and myristic acids.

Medium-chain fatty acids replacing tallow in milk replacers have been shown to result in increased protein and energy digestibility,[30] and to improve gain:feed ratios and reduce medical treatment costs.[31] Tallow or lard should be sourced as edible-grade fats fresh from the packing house, low in free fatty acids or with minimal peroxide values. Fats should be typical in color, taste, or smell and preserved with an antioxidant.

A blend of fats and oils can be successfully added to milk replacers in several ways. The most widely used is via blending liquid fats and oils with liquid whey, homogenizing to reduce and standardize the fat micron size to around 1 micron and then spray drying the liquid blend into a fat-filled powder typically composed of 7% to 10% protein and 50% to 60% fat. If properly manufactured the dry powder readily suspends in milk replacer solution. Also, the protein encapsulation does not break during routine CMR mixing and feeding procedures and at a robust range of temperatures.

In an improperly manufactured fat-filled powder, the protein encapsulation breaks and the fat spills out into the milk replacer solution. The fat then promptly separates out like cream, resulting, at best, into a greasy mess of milk mixing and feeding equipment, and, at worst, digestive disturbances in the calf. Care should be taken to not unnecessarily over-mix (avoid high-shear) milk replacer solution as this practice can break sensitive protein encapsulation in fat-filled powders.

A second means to administer fats and oils in milk replacers is with nonencapsulated blends. If administered into milk replacer powder properly, the liquid fat blend is crystalized using fast-freeze liquid nitrogen or CO_2 and the resulting finished powder flows and handles adequately for most climates and for most on-farm scenarios. These are known as free-fat systems as they lack protein encapsulation on the fat.

If administered on-farm, free fat is stored and applied as a liquid into the milk replacer solution. Whether freeze-crystalized at the milk replacer plant, or

Table 4
Milk-fed calf fat digestibility research examples

Fat or oil source	n	CMR Crude Fat (CF)%	CMR intake g/d	Age of calves (d)	% of Fat in CMR	Fat Digestibility (%)	Emulsifier	Grain Fed?	Citation
Crystalized fat (MSG; source N/A) whey diet	9	15.0%	1220	22–37	100%	90.4%	No	No	Ansia et al,[24] 2020. U of Illinois
Crystalized fat (MSG; source N/A) soy diet	9	15.0%	1240	22–37	100%	89.9%	No	No	
Palm oil (w/coconut oil, lecithin & emulsifier)	28	20.5%	N/R	app. 17	65%	96.9%	Yes	No (Veal)	Smink et al,[28] 2012. Wageningen NL
Tallow, homogenized & spray-dried w/skim milk; Skim milk diet.	6	20.8%	2309	77–141	100%	91.8%	Yes	No (Veal)	Toullec et al,[9] 1998. IN RA, France
Tallow, homogenized & spray dried in whey; High wheat (17.9%) formula	6	20.4%	2309	77–141	100%	93.6%	Yes	No (Veal)	[9]
Tallow, homogenized & spray dried in whey; lower wheat formula (9%)	6	20.6%	2309	77–141	100%	93.0%	Yes	No (Veal)	
Tallow, skim milk protein formula	7	20.2%	1090	39–44	98.5%	87.3%	No	No (Veal)	Lallés et al,[4] 1995. IN RA, France
Tallow, soy protein isolate formula	7	19.4%	1090	39–44	98.5%	89.5%	No	No (Veal)	[4]
Tallow, heated soy flour formula	7	20.0%	1090	39–44	98.5%	83.5%	No	No (Veal)	
Tallow in skim milk protein encapsulated fat	7	20.5%	1080	21–35	100.0%	91.7%	No	No (Veal)	Guilloteau et al,[29] 1986. IN RA, FR

Tallow in skim milk protein diet	8	22.6%	800–1400	13-	100%	93.7%	Yes	No (Veal)	Aurousseau et al,[30] 1984. IN RA, France
Tallow (1/3), Coconut (1/3), Tricaproin (1/3)	8	22.6%	800–1400	13-	Mix	97.3%	Yes	No (Veal)	[30]

Table 5
Typical fatty acid profile of fats and oils[33]

Fatty Acid	Chain length	Double Bonds	Butter	Lard	Tallow	Coconut	Palm Kernel oil	Palm oil	Soy oil	Canola oil	Veal Feed Fat
Butyric Acid	C4	0	4.5	<0.1	<0.1	<0.1	<0.1	<0.1	<0.1	<0.1	0
Caprylic acid	C8	0	1.4	<0.1	<0.1	0.8	4.1	<0.1	<0.1	<0.1	0.2
Capric acid	C1O	0	3.1	<0.1	0.1	6.2	3.6	<0.1	<0.1	<0.1	1.3
Laurie acid	C12	0	3.7	0.1	0.1	48.4	49.0	0.2	<0.1	<0.1	9.8
Myristic acid	C14	0	11.4	1.6	3.3	17.7	15.4	1	0.1	0.1	5.3
Palmitic acid	C16	0	29.8	27.1	27.4	8.4	8.3	44.5	10.7	4.5	21.3
Hexadecenoic acid	C16	1	2.2	2.2	3.0	<0.1	<0.1	0.2	0.1	0.2	1.9
Stearic acid	C18	0	10.1	18.5	23.2	2.5	2.1	4.4	4.3	1.6	15.5
Arachidic acid	C20	0	0.1	0.2	0.2	0.1	0.1	0.4	0.3	0.5	0.2
Tetradecenoic acid;	C14	1	1	0.1	0.5	<0.1	<0.1	<0.1	<0.1	<0.1	0.2
Oleic acid	C18	1	19.2	34.3	31.6	5.7	14.4	38.4	20.6	58	25.8
Linoleic acid	C18	2	1.5	9.9	1.8	1.4	2.3	9.5	53.7	20.5	4.5
Linoleic acid	C18	3	<0.1	<0.1	<0.1	<0.1	<0.1	<0.1	0.2	<0.1	0.0

administered as bulk liquid on-farm, free fat requires a proper emulsification system composed of an appropriate source and ratio of hydrophilic emulsifier and lecithin. An emulsification system is used both to stabilize the fat in the milk replacer solution (prevent creaming) and to improve nutrient digestibility in the calf. These systems have the disadvantage of providing a fat with a larger and more variable micron size, however, they also provide an emulsification system composed of hydrophilic emulsifiers shown to improve feed conversion and ADG.[32]

Both systems, free fat and encapsulated fat, have been shown to deliver excellent results if used within their mixing and feeding constraints. The constraint with a protein encapsulated fat is exposing the encapsulation to too much shear during the preparation of drink milk. The constraint with a free fat system is always maintaining proper minimum temperature so that your free fat does not crystallize resulting in fat separation.

Butterfat contains 4.5% butyric acid,[33] and all replacement fats and oils are void of butyric acid. Video 4 provides further information pertaining to the use of butyric acid in milk replacers.

VITAMINS AND MINERALS – CLINIC CARE POINTS

- Whole milk is deficient in most vitamins and all trace minerals.
- A subset of newborn calves is born anemic and requires iron supplementation. Anemia results in poor health and performance.
- Calves are born with low serum 25(OH)D concentrations and whole milk contain little vitamin D_3.
- Supplementing vitamins A, E, C, and D_3 have each been shown to improve calf health, growth, and/or immune function.
- Calves have a copper requirement; however, supplementation beyond NRC levels can be toxic. Excessive copper supplementation to the dam during gestation sets the calf up for toxicity.

A gallon of whole milk fails to meet NRC 2001 daily nutrient requirements for 7 essential trace minerals and all vitamins except vitamin A. These are established requirements for a healthy 45 kg (99 pounds) calf gaining 300 g per day (0.66 lb/d) (**Table 6**).

Anemia is a key concern because of milk's deficiencies. A calf is considered anemic if hemoglobin is less than 7.0 g/100 mL of blood and marginally anemic if between 7.0 and 7.9 g/100 mL.[35]

A survey of incoming veal calves (n = 757) conducted by Penn State University in 1999 found that 4.8% of calves were between 6.0 and 7.0 (anemic) and another 23% were between 7.0 and 8.9 g (a portion of these marginally anemic) of hemoglobin/100 mL of blood.[36] Veal farms typically procure the most robust calves thus the incidence of anemia is likely greater in the general dairy calf population.

A 2012 Iranian survey of 164 Holstein calves reared on 25 farms and fed whole milk perhaps captured a more realistic instance of anemia when the researchers reported a 17.7% incidence.[37]

Calves fed 10 mg rather than 50 mg of iron daily in the milk replacer noted poorer growth, poorer feed conversion, increased incidence of infections (particularly pneumonia), increased incidence of fever, more antibiotic treatments, poorer cell-mediated immunity, fewer neutrophils with phagocytic capacity, and lesser blood serum IgG concentration (all $P < .05$).[38] Milk-fed calves need supplemental iron.

Supplementing whole milk with vitamin E is shown to improve calf health and growth. One study noted reduced inflammation commonly associated with increased

Table 6
Vitamin and trace mineral requirements for the calf, nutrient concentrations in milk and Animix recommendations

Nutrient (Vitamin or T.M.)	A(IU)	D3(IU)	E(IU)	C (mg)	B1 (mg)	B2 (mg)	B3 (mg)	B6 (mg)	B5 (mg)	B12 (mog)	Biotin (mog)	B9 (mg)	Mn (mg)	Zn (mg)	Cu (mg)	Fe (mg)	CO (mg)	Se (mg)	I (mg)
Calf Requirement IU kg or ppm (NRC2001[26])	9000	600	50	0	6.5	6.5	10	6.5	13	70	100	0.5	40	40	10	100	0.11	0.3	0.5
Nutrient/gallon (3.8 L) of whole milk (NRC2001)	5216	139	3.6	MR	N/R	MR	N/R	N/R	N/R	N/R	N/R	N/R	0.13	12	0.27	1.4	0.002	0.04	0.07
Nutrients'/ Gallon 3.25% fat milk (USDA*)[27]	3593	1294*	2.5	MR	1.9	4.7	3.5	N/R	12.2	18.2	N/R	0	0	14.2	0.03	0	N/R	0.06	1.3
Animix Suggested fortification (IU/kg or ppm)	20,000	5000	100	300	13	13	20	13	26	65	90	8	40	40	10	100	0.11	0.3	0.5

Vitamin B1 - Thiamine	Vitamin B3- Niacin	Vitamin B6- Pyridoxine	* USDA Food Data Central for Milk, whole, 3.25% milk fat, w/added vitamin D[27]
Vitamin B2-Rboflavin	Vitamin B5- Pant. Acid	Vitamin B9- Folic acid	N/R = NOT REPORTED
			^ 530 g/d OMR, 45 kg BW, gaining 300 g/d (26)[34]

A gallon of whole milk fails to meet the calf's <u>trace mineral</u> requirements . . .

- Manganese – NRC requirement 18.1 mg. Provides 0.13 mg,^ 0.7% <u>of NRC</u>
- Zinc – NRC is 18.1 mg. Provides 12 mg,^ 66%.
- Copper – NRC is 4.53 mg. Provides 0.27 mg,^ 6%
- Iron – NRC 45.4 mg. Provides 1.2 mg,^ 2.6%
- Cobalt – NRC 0.05 mg. Provides 0.002 mg,^ 4%
- Selenium – NRC 0.13 mg. Provides 0.01 – 0.07 mg,^ 8 to 54%
- Iodine– NRC 0.23 mg. Provides 0.07 mg,^ 30%

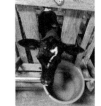

^ = NRC 2001. NRC reports no b-vitamin levels for whole milk
• = USDA FoodData Central for milk, whole, 3.25% milk fat, with added vitamin D3
https://fdc.nal.usda.gov/fdc-app.html#/food-details/746782/nutrients

Fig. 2. Trace mineral content of whole milk.

dietary energy intake ($P < .005$), a trend toward improved ADG ($P = .066$), and that serum α-tocopherol levels became more depleted with enhanced growth ($P < .05$), indicative of an increased vitamin E requirement associated with increased growth.[39] Supplementing 100 IU as compared with 20 IU of vitamin E daily resulted in improved ($P = .05$) ADG and reduced fecal scores ($P = .05$).[40]

Calves are born with just 15 ng/mL of serum 25(OH)D (vitamin D3) concentrations and remained near or less than 15 ng/mL through 1 month of life if fed unsupplemented whole milk and with little or no summer sun exposure.[41] Supplementing vitamin D3 at 5000 IU/d improved tolerance to an endotoxin challenge in calves as compared with supplementing NRC levels (600 IU/d).[42]

Excessive vitamin A (250,000 IU injection, plus daily supplementation of either 12,500 IU or 25,000 IU) supplementation to calves fed whole milk resulted in

A gallon of whole milk fails to meet the calf's <u>vitamin</u> requirements . . .

- Vitamin A – NRC requirement 4,770 IU. Provides 5216 IU,^ 109% of NRC
- Vitamin E – NRC is 26.5 IU. Provides 3.6 IU,^* 14% of NRC
- Vitamin D3 – NRC is 318 IU. Provides 139 IU^ or zero,* 0% to 44%
- B1, Thiamin – NRC is 3.45 mg. Provides 1.9 mg,* 55%
- B3, Niacin – NRC 5.3 mg. Provides 4 mg,* 75%
- B6, Pyridoxine – NRC 3.45 mg. Provides 1.6 mg,* 46%
- B12 – NRC 37.1 mcg. Provides 17.2 mcg,* 46%
- B9, Folic Acid – NRC 0.29 mg. Provides 0.2 mg,* 69%

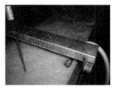

^ = NRC 2001. NRC reports no b-vitamin levels for whole milk
• * = USDA FoodData Central for milk, whole, 3.25% milk fat, with added vitamin D3
https://fdc.nal.usda.gov/fdc-app.html#/food-details/746782/nutrients

Fig. 3. Vitamin content of whole milk.

decreased (200 g/d) (0.44 lb/d) ($P < .05$) 0 to 3 weeks body weight gain.[43] Supplementing vitamin A at appropriate levels is shown to improve eye health (app. 16,000 IU daily) and reduce the incidence of diarrhea ($\geq$3000 IU/d).[44]

Videos 5–10 are supportive information pertaining to the effects of supplementing iron, vitamin E, vitamin D3, vitamin A, copper, and vitamin C, respectively, to the milk-fed calf, and **Figs. 2** and **3** show micronutrient contributions of whole milk.

Equal care should be given to meeting nutrient requirements and doing so using only wholesome, fresh, suitable ingredients. This is important both for milk replacer ingredients and when feeding whole milk. A survey conducted by Land O'Lakes of milk samples pre and postpasteurization from 618 farms noted a coefficient of variation for solids, fat, and protein of 6.58%, 7.9%, and 17.32% within a farm, respectively. This same field survey noted bacteria counts postpasteurization categorized as failed (>100,000 cfu), poor (20,001–100,000 cfu), or good ($\geq$20,000 cfu) occurring on 27.4%, 14.1%, and 58.4% of farms, respectively.[45]

SUMMARY

Protein (amino acid), fat (fatty acid), carbohydrate (lactose), mineral, and vitamin requirements necessary for maintaining health and meeting growth goals should be met by offering the calf wholesome, suitable sources. Care should be taken to ensure these requirements are met whether the farm offers the calf whole milk, milk replacer as a complete powder or assembled from components on farm, or a mixture of all 3. Equal scrutiny on suitability should be administered on all nutritional components of the liquid diet, including on-farm derived whole milk. Bovine practitioners can play a key role in ensuring sound consistent wholesome nutrition occurs for the milk-fed calf.

DISCLOSURE

Animix provides as either ingredients or premixes all AAFCO-approved micronutrients and feed additives milk replacer customers require including specialized water-dispersible vitamins, minerals, spray-dried plasma proteins, hydrolyzed wheat protein, emulsifiers and spray drying aids. Animix markets products to milk replacer manufacturers primarily in N. America but also around the world.

ACKNOWLEDGMENTS

The lipids section was reviewed, and valued input was provided by Bert Wijnholds M Sci. and Jeroen van Roon Ph.D. of Functional Solutions, Agro Business Park 62, 6708 PW Wageningen, Netherlands. Functional Solutions provides emulsifiers and spray drying aids and valued advice on lipids to the veal feed and milk replacer industries. All sections were reviewed, and input was provided by Ronelle Blome M.S., calf nutritionist and executive V.P. of Animix, Juneau, WI.

SUPPLEMENTARY DATA

Supplementary data related to this article can be found online at https://doi.org/10.1016/j.cvfa.2021.11.01.

REFERENCES

1. Thornsberry RM, Wood D, Kertz AF, et al. Alternative ingredients in calf milk replacer – a review for bovine practitioners. Bov Pract 2016;50:65–88. https://doi.org/10.21423/bovine-vol50no1p65-88. Available at:.

2. Grongnet JF, Patureau-Mirand P, Toullec R, et al. Utilisation des protéins du lait et du lactosérum par le jeune veau préruminant. Influence de l'age et de la dénaturation des protéins du lactosérum. Ann Zootech 1981;30:443–64.

3. Dawson DP, Morrill JL, Reddy PG, et al. Soy protein concentrate and heated soy flours as protein sources in milk replacer for preruminant calves. J Dairy Sci 1988; 71:1301–9. https://doi.org/10.3168/jds.S0022-0302(88)79687-3. Available at:.

4. Lallés JP, Toullec R, Branco Pardal P, et al. Hydrolyzed soy protein isolate sustains high nutritional performance in veal calves. J Dairy Sci 1995;78:194–204. https://doi.org/10.3168/jds.S0022-0302(95)76629-2. Available at:.

5. Liang Y, Carroll JA, Ballou MA, et al. The digestive system of 1-week-old Jersey calves is well suited to digest, absorb, and incorporate protein and energy into tissue growth even when calves are fed a high plane of milk replacer. J Dairy Sci 2016;99:1929–37. https://doi.org/10.3168/jds.2015-9895. Available at:.

6. Strudsholm F. The effect of curd formation in the abomasum on the digestion of milk replacers in preruminant calves. Acta Agric Scand 1988;38:321–7.

7. Terosky JL, Heinrichs AJ, Wilson LL, et al. A comparison of milk protein sources in diets of calves up to eight weeks of age. J Dairy Sci 1997;80:2977–83. https://doi.org/10.3168/jds.S0022-0302(97)76264-7. Available at:.

8. Tolman GH, Demeersman M. Digestibility and growth performance of soluble wheat protein for veal calves. In: Metz JHM, Groenestein CM, editors. New trends in veal calf production, EAAP Publication No. 52. Wageningen, Netherlands: Pudoc; 1991. p. 227–33.

9. Toullec R, Formal M. Digestion of wheat protein in the preruminant calf: ileal digestibility and blood concentrations of nutrients. Anim Feed Sci Tech 1998;73: 115–30. https://doi.org/10.1016/S0377-8401(98)00126-6. Available at:.

10. Besser TE, McQuire TC, Gay CC, et al. Transfer of functional immunoglobulin G (IgG) antibody into the gastrointestinal tract accounts for IgG clearance in calves. J Virol 1988;62:2234–7. https://doi.org/10.1128/jvi.62.7.2234-2237.1988. Available at:.

11. Pyo J, Hare K, Pletts S, et al. Feeding colostrum or a 1:1 colostrum:milk mixture for 3 days postnatal increases small intestinal development and minimally influences plasma glucagon-like peptide-2 and serum insulin-like growth factor-1 concentrations in Holstein bull calves. J Dairy Sci 2020;103:4236–51. https://doi.org/10.3168/jds.2019-17219. Available at:.

12. Bühler C, Hammon H, Giovanni LR, et al. Small intestinal morphology in eight-day-old calves fed colostrum for different durations or only milk replacer and treated with long-R^3-insulin-like growth factor I and growth hormone. J Anim Sci 1998;76:758–65. https://doi.org/10.2527/1998.763758x. Available at:.

13. Berge ACB, Besser TE, Moore DA, et al. Evaluation of the effects of oral colostrum supplementation during the first fourteen days on the health and performance of preweaned calves. J Dairy Sci 2009;92:286–95.

14. Nollet H, Laevens H, Deprez P, et al. The use of non-immune plasma powder in the prophylaxis of neonatal Escherichia coli diarrhea in calves. Am J Vet Med 1999;46:185–96. https://doi.org/10.1046/j.1439-0442.1999.00208.x. Available at:.

15. Quigley JD, Drew MD. Effects of oral antibiotics or bovine plasma on survival, health and growth in dairy calves challenged with Escherichia coli. Food Ag Immunol 2000;12:311–8.

16. Arthington JD, Jaynes CA, Tyler HD, et al. The use of bovine serum protein as an oral support therapy following coronavirus challenge in calves. J Dairy Sci 2002; 85:1249–54. https://doi.org/10.3168/jds.S0022-0302(02)74189-1. Available at:.

17. Hunt E, Qiang F, Armstrong M, et al. Oral bovine serum concentrate improves cryptosporidial enteritis in calves. Pediatr Res 2002;51:370–6. https://doi.org/10.1203/00006450-200203000-00017. Available at:.

18. Roos N, Mahe S, Benemouzig R, et al. 15N-labeled immunoglobulins from bovine colostrum are partially resistant to digestion in human intestine. J Nutr 1995;125:1238–44. https://doi.org/10.1093/jn/125.5.1238. Available at:.

19. Claxton R. Global veal market overview presentation: 5th International Veal Congress Proceedings. Gira Consultancy and Research Prospective et Strategic. Total European veal marketed: 5.8 million. May 19, 2011, Amsterdam, the Netherlands.

20. Grice KD, Glosson KM, Drackley JK, et al. Effects of feeding frequency and protein source in milk replacer for Holstein calves. J Dairy Sci 2020;103:10048–59. https://doi.org/10.3168/jds.2020-19041. Available at:.

22. Lallés JP, Tukur HM, Toullec R, et al. Analytical criteria for predicting apparent digestibility of soybean protein in preruminant calves. J Dairy Sci 1996;79:475–84. https://doi.org/10.3168/jds.S0022-0302(96)76388-9. Available at:.

21. Hill TM, Bateman HG, Aldrich JM, et al. Use of plasma, hydrolyzed wheat gluten, or the combination in dairy calf milk replacers. J Dairy Sci 2013;96(E-Suppl. 1):656.

23. Seegraber FJ, Morrill JL. Effect of protein source in calf milk replacers on morphology and absorptive ability of small intestine. J Dairy Sci 1985;69:460–9. https://doi.org/10.3168/jds.S0022-0302(86)80424-6. Available at:.

24. Ansia I, Stein HH, Vermeire DA, et al. Ileal digestibility and endogenous protein losses of milk replacers based on whey protein alone or with an enzyme-treated soybean meal in young dairy calves. J Dairy Sci 2020;103:4390–407. https://doi.org/10.3168/jds.2019-17699. Available at:.

25. Siddons RC. Carbohydrase activities in the bovine digestive tract. Biochem J 1968;108:839–44. https://doi.org/10.1042/bj1080839. Available at:.

26. Trotta RJ, Ward AK, Swanson KC, et al. Influence of dietary fructose supplementation on visceral organ mass, carbohydrase activity, and mRNA expression of genes involved in small intestinal carbohydrate assimilation in neonatal calves. J Dairy Sci 2020;103:10060–73. https://doi.org/10.3168/jds.2020-18145. Available at:.

27. USDA nutrient content of milk, whole, 3.25% milkfat, with added vitamin D. U.S. Department of Agriculture, Agricultural Research Service. Available at: https://fdc.nal.usda.gov/fdc-app.html#/food-details/746782/nutrients. Accessed May 25, 2021.

28. Smink W. Fatty acid digestion, synthesis and metabolism in broiler chickens and pigs. Neth J Agr Sci 2012. Available at: https://edepot.wur.nl/222198.

29. Guilloteau P, Toullec R, Grongnet JF, et al. Digestion of milk, fish, and soya-bean protein in the preruminant calf: flow of digesta, apparent digestibility at the end of the ileum and amino acid composition of ileal digesta. Br J Nutr 1986;55:571–92. https://doi.org/10.1079/BJN19860063. Available at:.

30. Aurousseau B, Vermorel M, Bouvier JC, et al. Influence du remplacement d'une partie du suif d'un aliment d'allaitement par de la tricapryline ou de l'huile de coprah sur l'utilisation de l'énergie et de l'azote par le veau préruminant. Reprod Nutr Develop 1984;24(3):265–79.

31. Ziegler D, Chester-Jones H, Ziegler B, et al. Performance and health of dairy calves fed milk replacers on a conventional or accelerated feeding rate supplemented with different fat sources. J Dairy Sci 2019;102(Suppl. 1).

32. Reis ME, Toledo AF, da Silva AP, et al. Supplementation of lysolecithin in milk replacer for Holstein dairy calves: Effects on growth performance, health, and metabolites. J Dairy Sci 2021;104:5457–66. https://doi.org/10.3168/jds.2020-19406. Available at:.

33. Hulshof PJM. Fatty acid composition of selected edible fats and oils. Wageningen, The Netherlands: Wageningen University; 2019. Available at: https://mvo.nl/media/report_fatty_acid_composition_of_selected_fats_and_oils_2019.pdf.

34. NRC. Nutrient requirements of dairy cattle. 7th Revised Edition, Subcommittee on dairy Cattle nutrition, Committee on animal nutrition, board on Agriculture and natural Resources. Washington, D.C: National Research Council, National Academy Press; 2001.

35. Schalm OW, Jain IC, Carroll EJ, et al. Veterinary Hematology. 3rd edition. Philadelphia, PA: Lea and Febiger; 1975.

36. Wilson LL, Smith JL, Smith DL, et al. Characteristics of veal calves upon arrival at 28 and 84 days, and at end of the production cycle. J Dairy Sci 2000. https://doi.org/10.3168/jds.S0022-0302(00)74948-4. Available at:.

37. Ramin AG, Siamak AR, Khales P, et al. Evaluation of anemia in calves up to 4 months of age in Holstein dairy herds. VETSCAN 2012;7:87–92.

38. Gygax M, Hirni H, Wahlen RZ, et al. Immune functions of veal calves fed low amounts of iron. J Vet Med A 1993;40:1–10.

39. Krueger LA, Beitz DC, Onda K, et al. Effects of d-α-tocopherol and dietary energy on growth and health of preruminant dairy calves. J Dairy Sci 2014;97:3715–27. https://doi.org/10.3168/jds.2013-7315. Available at:.

40. Luhman CM, Miller BL, Perry HB, et al. The effect of vitamin E addition on calves fed calf milk replacer. J Dairy Sci 1993;104(9):9769–83.

41. Nelson CD, Lippolis JD, Reinhardt TA, et al. Vitamin D status of dairy cattle: outcomes of current practices in the dairy industry. J Dairy Sci 2016;99:10150–60. https://doi.org/10.3168/jds.2016-11727. Available at:.

42. Buoniconti SM, Blakely LP, Reese M, et al. Effects of feeding 25-hydroxyvitamin D_3 to dairy calves: effects on responses to endotoxin challenge. J Dairy Sci 2019;102(Suppl. 1).

43. Blakely L, Kweb M, Poindexter M, et al. Effects of supplementing pasteurized waste milk with vitamins A, D, and E on fat soluble vitamin status, growth, and health of calves. J Dairy Sci 2016;99.

44. Eaton HD, Rousseau JE, Hall RC, et al. Reevaluation of the minimum vitamin A requirement of the Holstein male calves based upon elevated cerebrospinal fluid pressure. J Dairy Sci 1971;55:232–7. https://doi.org/10.3168/jds.S0022-0302(72)85465-1. Available at:.

45. Yoho WSB, Hansen CM, Stephas EL, et al. Variation of nutrient content and bacteria count of pasteurized waste milk fed to dairy calves. J Dairy Sci 2017;100(Suppl. 2).

Rumen Transition from Weaning to 400 Pounds

Randy W. Rosenboom, MS

KEYWORDS

- Rumen development • Weaned calf • Rumen papillae • Ruminal VFA production

KEY POINTS

- Rumen size changes dramatically from weaning 200 pounds (91 kg) to 400 pounds (181.8 kg) body weight.
- Rumen substrate is very influential to rumen development.
- Rumen papillae development is most important to rumen nutrient absorption.
- Grain is superior to forage in developing rumen papillae.
- Rumen size does not indicate papillae development.

INTRODUCTION

The average age at weaning in the United States is 9 weeks.[1] The actual age at cessation of milk feeding may be anywhere from 6 to 8 weeks, but the act of weaning usually implies a departure from the "nursery" facility and into a facility with small 8- to 12-head groups. Although the purpose of this article evaluates nutritional management to optimize rumen development, the importance of group size management to reduce stress and the incidence of bovine respiratory disease at weaning cannot be over emphasized. An 8- to 12-head group is ideal,[2,3] but groups of 20 weaned calves can be managed if pen space, bunk space, and water availability are optimal. An artfully formulated nutrition program cannot overcome poor management decisions. Water intake management is crucial to rumen development and fermentation.[4] Weaned calves have experienced individual feeding with a bucket of water and feed available to them at all times. They will be placed into a group pen with an automatic waterer they have never used and may not be able to locate. Some sort of supplemental water supply, such as an in-pen open top tank, is advisable until all the calves are consuming water.

PROMOTING RUMEN PAPILLAE DEVELOPMENT

The preweaning feeding program is important to create ideal rumen papillae development,[5,6] as illustrated by these photos from Penn State University[7] (**Figs. 1–3**). Calves

Kent Nutrition Group, 3363 170th Street, Estherville, IA 51334, USA
E-mail address: Randy.Rosenboom@kentww.com

Vet Clin Food Anim 38 (2022) 153–164
https://doi.org/10.1016/j.cvfa.2021.11.010
0749-0720/22/© 2021 Elsevier Inc. All rights reserved.

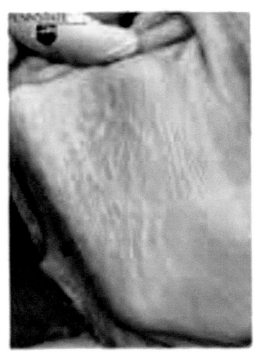

Fig. 1. Impact of preweaning diet composition on rumen papillae development. (Photos courtesy of Penn State Extension.)

fed milk or milk replacer as the sole diet and calves fed milk or milk replacer with hay do not develop rumen papillae quickly. Calves fed milk or milk replacers, with a starter feed, do develop rumen papillae, and they do so by 4 weeks of age. **Fig. 3** is a photograph of a 4-week-old calf rumen with good rumen papillae development, whereas **Figs. 1** and **2** are photographs of 12-week-old rumens with little to no rumen papillae development. Diet composition is important to rumen papillae development.

RUMEN SUBSTRATE EFFECT ON RUMEN DEVELOPMENT

Preweaning grain intake produces development of the rumen papillae.[8] There is a misconception that calves should be offered hay during preweaning management. Although the volume of the rumen as a percent of the 4 stomach compartments is essentially doubled by 8 weeks (**Table 1**), most rumen papillae development is a direct result of preweaning grain intake.[8] Adding a source of dietary structural carbohydrates into the preweaning diet limits rumen papillae growth and density.[9]

Preweaning rumen papillae growth and development determines the health of the rumen as well as the efficiency of rumen fermentation postweaning. A functional rumen at 8 weeks of age has volume limitations in providing for optimal and economic growth of the calf. It takes 2 to 4 weeks for specific classes of bacteria to populate the rumen and begin to efficiently ferment the structural carbohydrates in hay.[10] Research has demonstrated that diets can be fed containing 0%, 7.5%, and 15% of the dry matter diet as processed roughage in light calves.[11] However, this research controlled particle size, offering a smaller particle size (0.3–0.75 inches or 8–19 mm) than what

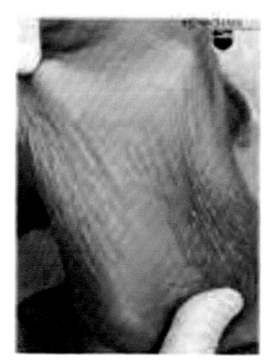

Fig. 2. Impact of preweaning diet composition on rumen papillae development. (Photos courtesy of Penn State Extension.)

is provided to most calves through 400 pounds (181.8 kg) in the field. This particle size would need less further mastication to provide adequate surface area for bacterial fermentation. These researchers proved that coarse grain was superior to ground grain with regard to all rumen characteristics and volatile fatty acid (VFA) production. They also concluded that butyrate and propionate were superior to acetate for papillae growth, which supports a preference for a grain-based as opposed to a forage-based diet.

RUMEN VOLUME AND ESTIMATED INTAKE

Assuming a rumen volume illustration of 1 gallon (3.79 L), this volume can accommodate 6 pounds (2.73 kg) of grain mix or 1 pound (.45 kg) of hay. The potential energy availability difference between these 2 feedstuffs is obvious simply due to rumen volume limitations. Butyrate and propionate are the primary VFAs produced from grain. Acetate is the primary VFA produced from hay. Acetate retards rumen papillae growth and development, giving a significant advantage in rumen fill volume to a grain-based diet for preweaned and postweaned calves. Rumen papillae length is considered the most important factor to rumen development in small ruminants.[12]

It is appropriate to feed as much grain mix as the calves will eat preweaning and postweaning. In general, around 3% of body weight on an as-fed basis is provided each day. For dairy beef calves, maintain the level of intake through 400 pounds (181.8 kg) of body weight. Replacement dairy heifers are limit fed to produce 2 to 2.5 pounds (0.91–1.14 kg) of body weight gain per day. A small amount of high-

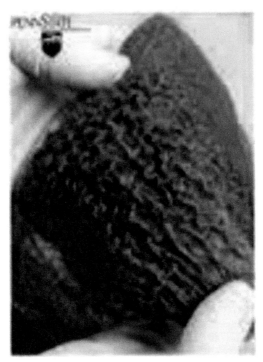

Fig. 3. Impact of preweaning diet composition on rumen papillae development. (Photos courtesy of Penn State Extension.)

quality roughage is provided around 300 to 350 pounds (136.4–159 kg) of body weight. When replacement dairy heifers reach 400 pounds (181.8 kg), moderate the energy levels in their diets to avoid excessive fat deposition in the udder. The goal is to manage replacement dairy heifer diets to produce adequate daily gain without depositing excess body fat. Monitoring dry matter intake for replacement dairy heifers to include higher roughage levels is a good indicator of diet adequacy. Adapting to fiber first and then introducing ensiled feedstuffs, preferably after 400 pounds (181.8 kg) body weight, is recommended. As always, evaluating weight and hip height appropriateness for age is crucial. A more detailed discussion of proper diet transition procedure from all grain diets to an age-appropriate total mixed ration (TMR) for these light calves is presented in another section of this article.

Table 1			
Impact of age on percent volume of stomach compartments			
%	0 wk	8 wk	12 wk
Reticulorumen	38.0	61.2	67.0
Omasum	13.0	13.4	18.0
Abomasum	49.0	25.4	15.0

From Review of strategies to promote rumen development in calves. *Animal* 9 (8): 490; Diao, Zhang and Fu. 2019

Table 2
Effect of percent hay in dry matter diet on performance of 12-week-old calves

Concentrate lb/d	1	2	3	4	5
% Hay DMB	61	31	28	16	4
ADG lb/d	.70	.92	1.03	1.32	1.30
Live wt lb/hd	130	139	132	172	170
Rumen papillae, mm	4.2	5.2	5.5	7.4	7.4
% of Live Weight					
Reticulorumen	18	15	14	11	10
Alimentary tract	23	20	19	15	14

Abbreviation: DMB, dry matter basis,

DIET COMPOSITION EFFECT ON PERFORMANCE AND RUMEN PARAMETERS IN LIGHT CALVES

Much of the research done on immature rumen development was published in the 1950s and 60s.[13–17] It is warranted to refresh the data set with today's genetics and additives that may alter some of these tried and true principles.[18]

A. F. Kertz presented a concise summary of some of this historical research in an article in Progressive Dairy, January 13, 2021.[19] He referenced published peer-reviewed research that concluded grain intake stimulates rumen papillae development, and the scratch factor of fiber feeds may increase rumen size, but does little to increase papillae, and therefore nutrient absorption, in ruminants up to 12 weeks of age. The following is a summary table he referenced in this article (**Table 2**).

There was a question raised by Dr Kertz regarding gut fill. For calves this small with this wide variation in hay intake, the influence of gut fill probably makes the true body weight and corresponding average daily gain differences even greater. In future research, an attempt to correct for this factor should be considered.

ANECDOTAL PRESENTATION OF ACTUAL PERFORMANCE IN A COMMERCIAL CALF GROWER OPERATION

The following is a summary of 2 years of calf ranch data, collected from the field by this investigator. The field study facility is a well-managed operation that uses a whole-grain, coarse grain program with no hay feeding. The only roughage intake is from the bedding in the barns. This bedding was run through a forage processer so its utilization may support previous reported forage processing research.[11] Each year represents 5 groups of 340 hutch calves from weaning, 9 weeks, to 400 pounds (181.8 kg) (**Table 3**).

These data are presented to allow for economic analysis for current ingredient costs of this high-grain diet versus a lower cost, high-roughage diet. Once calves reach this

Table 3
Two year's calf ranch summary performance data (9 weeks to 400 pounds)

Head In	Head Out	In Wt	Out Wt	DOF	ADG	F/G	Daily Feed
1680	1676	209	416	68	3.05	3.26	9.93
1673	1668	201	423	71	3.13	3.27	10.26

Abbreviations: DOF, days on feed; ADG, average daily gain; F/G, feed to gain ratio.
  All units in pounds; daily feed-as fed.

stage, rumen development is complete, and the attending nutritionist is tasked with formulating diets that promote optimal rumen microbe populations, balanced against the economies of feeding cattle.

EXAMPLE DIETS AND TRANSITION STRATEGIES FOR YOUNG RUMINANTS

Table 4 illustrates 2 grain mixes composed of whole corn and a commercial protein supplement pellet. The mix containing 600 pounds (272.7 kg) of pellets and 1400 pounds (636.4 kg) of whole corn is for calves weighing 200 to 250 pounds (113.6–159 kg). The mix containing 500 pounds (227.3 kg) of pellets and 1500 pounds (681.8 kg) of whole corn is for calves weighing 250 to 350 pounds (113.6–159 kg). As mentioned previously, the intakes are approximately 3% of body weight as fed.

There is a much more detailed nutrient analysis available, but it is not pertinent to this consideration. Dry matter, protein, and Net Energy (NEm [maintenance] and NEg [gain]) are the primary considerations in proper ration transition for rumen stability. The macro- and microminerals as well as vitamins are balanced to meet or exceed National Research Council requirements.[20]

To illustrate the 3% of body weight as-fed intake, a 250 pounds (113.6 kg) calf will consume approximately 2.5% of its body weight on a dry matter basis each day. Therefore, 250 pounds (113.6 kg) X .025 = 6.25 pounds (2.84 kg) of dry matter. Next, divide 6.25 pounds (2.84 kg) dry matter by 86% dry matter in the diet, which yields 7.26 pounds (3.3 kg) as fed. The same procedure can be applied to each weight break of diet assignment. Most of these calves are fed in well-bedded barns where bedding intake prepares the rumen to begin developing bacteria that digest fiber. As the calf intake grows, this moderate amount of fiber digesting bacteria helps promote a stable rumen with regard to pH. The dietary management of calves housed in facilities without bedding, that is, slatted floors or sawdust or sand bedding, present a challenge, as fiber will need to be incorporated in the diet formulation. Processed hay or straw at 7.5% to 15% of the diet should be considered.[11]

TRANSITION STRATEGY FROM A GRAIN MIX TO A TOTAL MIXED RATION

Shown here are 3 TMRs to transition calves from the grain mix to a TMR. The first TMR is to accustom the calf to a higher moisture diet as well as another protein and energy

Table 4
Two age-specific grain-based diets, whole corn/commercial pellet (32% protein) grain mix expressed in pounds per ton

Ingredient	200–250 pounds Body Wt	250–350 pounds Body Wt
Whole corn	1400	1500
32% CP pellet	600	500
Nutrient Analysis (Dry Matter %)		
Dry matter%	86.50	86.25
Crude protein%	16.60	15.19
Crude fat%	3.12	3.24
NEm Mcal/cwt	93.82	95.10
NEg Mcal/cwt	63.62	64.72
Ca %	.89	.75
P %	.56	.52

Table 5
Formulations for a total mixed ration feeding program in percentages of total diet

Ingredient	TMR 1	TMR 2	TMR 3
Balancer	1.55	1.60	1.48
Grass hay	12.72	8.83	.60
Corn silage			25.00
Cracked corn	43.91	28.23	28.73
High-moisture ear corn		25.00	14.36
Modified distillers grain	41.82	36.34	29.83
Nutrient Analysis (DM%)			
Dry matter %	68.27	67.27	58.84
Crude protein %	14.00	13.50	13.00
Crude fat %	4.53	4.36	4.39
NEm mcal/cwt	93.10	92.24	94.63
NEg mcal/cwt	63.00	63.00	65.00
Calcium %	.60	.60	.60
Phosphorus %	.40	.38	.37

source as provided by the distiller's grain (modified distiller's grain is approximately 45% dry matter). The second TMR introduces an ensiled feedstuff, high-moisture ear corn; this provides a similar energy and protein level as TMR 1 but presents a lower pH feedstuff to the rumen microbes. The third TMR introduces another ensiled feedstuff, corn silage, which adapts the developing rumen to higher moisture and higher volume feedstuffs (**Table 5**).

A simple strategy to transition a calf from a grain mix to a TMR is shown here. The percentages are on an as-fed basis (**Table 6**).

As the calves are transitioned to the TMR, be mindful that 2.5% of the calf's body weight is a target for dry matter intake. To commence the transition, the calves should weigh 350 pounds (159 kg). If they are to consume 2.5% of their body weight on a dry matter basis, it translates into 8.75 pounds (3.98 kg). If an all-grain mix is fed, that would be 8.75 divided by 86% equaling 10.2 pounds (4.64 kg) as fed. Multiply 10.2 pounds (4.64 kg) X 75% to obtain 7.7 pounds (3.5 kg) of grain mix for step 1. If all the 8.75 pounds (3.98 kg) dry matter came from the TMR 1, divide 8.75 by 68% and obtain 12.9 pounds (5.86 kg) as fed. Multiply 12.9 pounds (5.86 kg) X 25% and obtain 3.2 pounds (1.45 kg) as fed; this may seem confusing at first, but after doing multiple calculations and correlating dry matter intake to "as fed" intake, it becomes understandable. Once the calves are completely on TMR 1, they will probably be about 400 pounds (181.8 kg) and eating 15 pounds (6.82 kg) of the TMR as fed. That is 400 pounds (181.8 kg) X 2.5% = 10 pounds (4.54 kg) dry matter. Divide 10 pounds (4.54 kg) dry matter by 68% to obtain 14.7 pounds (6.68 kg) as fed. The TMR 2 is to introduce the calves to an ensiled feedstuff, high-moisture ear corn. This TMR could be started once the calves weigh 475 to 500 pounds (216–227.3 kg) and fed until they weigh approximately 600 pounds (272.7 kg). At that time, they should be capable of eating approximately 28 pounds (12.7 kg) as fed of TMR 3. This diet can be fed until market weight. This assumes the calves are dairy or dairy crossbred calves. If the calves are straight beef calves, a different diet sequence may need to be implemented from 300 pounds (136.4 kg) body weight.

Table 6
Transition from dry grain–based ration to total mixed ration, percent of diet as fed

	Day 1–5	Day 6–10	Day 11–15
Grain mix	75%	50%	25%
TMR 1	25%	50%	75%

GROWER RATION STRATEGY FOR LIGHTWEIGHT REPLACEMENT HEIFERS

The following is a ration that is being used for dairy replacement heifers in a current facility. There are literally dozens of diet compositions that can be formulated, but this illustrates an example of what can be successfully fed to 400 pound (181.8 kg) dairy heifers that are being developed to 600 pounds (272.7 kg) before going to another facility where they will be grown and bred; this supports a growth rate of approximately 2.5 lb/d (1.14 kg/d) (**Table 7**).

It is important, when feeding lightweight, immature ruminants, to evaluate body condition and monitor dry matter intake. This monitoring, plus fecal consistency observations, will give an external indication of how well the rumen biome is adapting to the diet changes. During the stage from 200 to 400 pounds (91–181.8 kg) body weight, it is advisable to make daily dry matter intake increases of 0.5 to 0.75 pounds (0.22–0.34 kg) DM/head/day. Once an increase has been made, wait 3 to 4 days to make another increase and evaluate fecal consistency daily.

Stools from a calf with a well-adapted rumen should be light gold to light yellow with a formed pile that has a stiff pudding consistency (**Fig. 4**). If stools puddle out, or are watery, then the rumen is undergoing subclinical to clinical acidosis (**Figs. 5** and **6**).

Transit time from feed ingestion until it is completely out of the rumen is 35 to 48 hours but varies with the forage to concentrate ratio and the daily dry matter intake.[21] This is a continuum with portions of the feed passing out while new ingesta

Table 7
Replacement heifer total mixed ration fed from 400 to 600 pounds (ingredients expressed on a percent as-fed basis)

Ingredient	Replacement Heifer Diet
Grass hay	7.20
Corn silage	46.00
Cracked corn	9.00
Oats	20.00
Modified distiller's grain	15.00
Commercial 45% CP supplement	2.8
Nutrient analysis (DM)	
DM %	56.88
Crude protein %	13.80
Crude fat %	4.23
NEm mcal/lb	80.13
NEg mcal/lb	53.62
Calcium %	.63
Phosphorous	.39

Abbreviation: DM, dry matter.

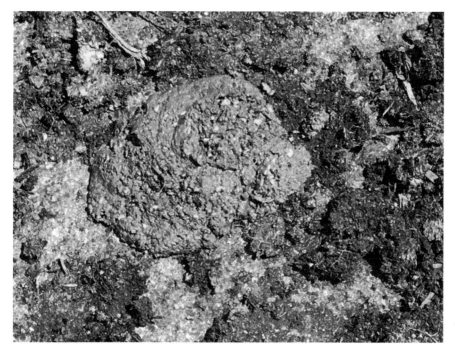

Fig. 4. Stool that indicates a well-adapted rumen.

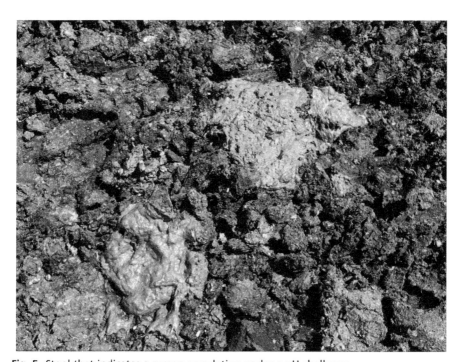

Fig. 5. Stool that indicates a rumen population under a pH challenge.

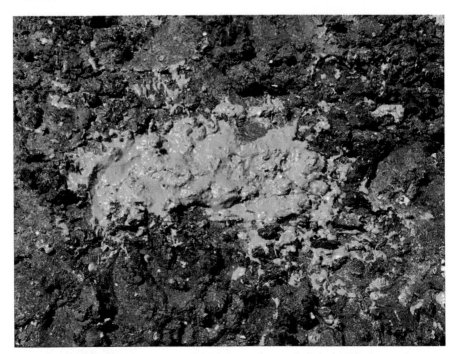

Fig. 6. Stool that indicates a rumen undergoing at least subclinical acidosis.

enter the alimentary tract and is significant when evaluating manure quality. If stools are loose, the intake event or ration change that caused it probably happened 2 to 3 days before the loose stools present. The looseness is caused by water being drawn into the digestive tract by osmosis due to fermentation products in the lumen of the intestinal tract. This is the response of the digestive tract to a nutritional insult.[22] This event, combined with an increased rate of passage, is how the digestive tract responds to rumen acidosis. From a management standpoint, keeping calves well bedded is important. It is impossible to implement a diet change to accommodate a small percentage of calves in a group with rumen acidosis. If clean dry bedding is accessible at all times, the animal can consume some fiber, which will generate saliva from mastication and help buffer the rumen.[22]

Weather events can trigger cattle to overconsume an available ration. Because cattle are usually fed in groups, it is difficult to observe which individuals have overconsumed their ration until the loose stools present. Looseness can also be triggered by offering more feed than the rumen is capable of fermenting or making an increase in energy too quickly or too great in magnitude. Increasing cattle 1 pound of dry matter (.454 kg) is the same as moving it up by 3 mcal NEg/100 pounds (45.45 kg) in a diet sequence. Making daily DM increases of no more than 1 lb/d (.454 kg) and then waiting 3 to 5 days before making another is advisable. It is also a good practice to increase NEg by no more than 3 mcal/100 pounds (45.45 kg) between diet changes. That is why animal and fecal consistency observation is critical to the management of a successful dietary regimen.

SUMMARY

Rumen development in young calves, 8 weeks to 400 pounds (181.8 kg), will be most successful if the first diet consumed promotes rumen papillae growth. This requires a diet that promotes butyric and propionic acid production. Grain-based diets promote butyrate and propionate production, whereas forage-based diets promote acetate production. When the calf reaches 350 pounds (159 kg), additional protein sources and higher moisture feeds, such as modified distiller's grains, can be introduced to the diet. As dry matter intakes build and the calf matures, ensiled feedstuffs such as high-moisture ear corn can be introduced. And finally, the next step to diet sequencing is to introduce a high-moisture, high-volume feedstuff, such as corn silage to the diet. Observing manure quality and consistency is an important tool to evaluate rumen microflora adaptation to diet changes. Be mindful that it may take up to 48 hours for a complete rumen turn over regarding daily feed intake. Degradation in stool quality can be the result of an event or nutritional insult that took place 24 to 48 hours before the stool change presents.

DISCLOSURE

The author has nothing to disclose.

REFERENCES

1. USDA. 2018. Dairy 2014, Health and Management Practices on U.S. Dairy Operations, 2014. USDA-Animal and Plant Health Inspection Service-Veterinary Services-Center for Epidemiology and Animal Health-National Animal Health Monitoring System (USDAAPHIS-VS-CEAH-NAHMS), Fort Collins, CO. Fort Collins, CO. #696.0218.
2. Gulliksen SM, Jor E, Lie KI, et al. Respiratory infections in Norwegian dairy calves. J Dairy Sci 2009a;92:5139–46.
3. Gulliksen SM, Lie KI, Loken T, et al. Calf mortality in Norwegian dairy herds. J Dairy Sci 2009b;92:2782–95.
4. Kertz AF, Reutzel LF, Mahoney JH. Ad libitum water intake by neonatal calves and its relationship to calf starter intake, weight gain, feces score, and season. J Dairy Sci 1984;67:2964–9.
5. Hill TM, Bateman HG II, Aldrich JM, et al. Methods of reducing milk replacer to prepare dairy calves for weaning when large amounts of milk replacer have been fed. Prof Anim Sci 2012;28:332–7.
6. Steele MA, Doelman JH, Leal LN, et al. Abrupt weaning reduces postweaning growth and is associated with alterations in gastrointestinal markers of development in dairy calves fed an elevated plane of nutrition during the preweaning period. J Dairy Sci 2017;100:5390–9.
7. Penn State Extension. Available at: www.extension.psu.edu/photos-of-rumen-development.
8. Zitman R, Voigt J, Schonhusen U, et al. Influence of dietary concentrate to forage ratio on the development of rumen mucosa in calves. Arch Tierernahr 1998;51(4):279–91.
9. Available at: www.ndvsu.org/images/StudyMaterials/Nutrition/FEEDING-OF-CALVES.pdf. Slide 9.
10. Dias Juliana, Inácio Marcondes Marcos, Motta de Souza Shirley, et al. Bacterial Community Dynamics across the Gastrointestinal Tracts of Dairy Calves during Preweaning Development. Appl Environ Microbiol 2018;84(9):e02675–026717.
11. Coverdale JA, Tyler HD, Quigley JD, et al. Effect of various levels of forage and form of diet on rumen development and growth in calves. J Dairy Sci 2004;87(8):2554–62.
12. Lesmeister RE, Tozer PR, Heinrichs AJ. Development and analysis of a rumen tissue sampling procedure. J Dairy Sci 2004;87(5):1336–44.

13. Flatt WP, Warner RG, Loosli JK. Influence of purified materials on the development of the ruminant stomach. J Dairy Sci 1958;41:1593–600.
14. Sander EG, Warner RG, Harrison HN, et al. The stimulatory effect of sodium butyrate and sodium propionate on the development of rumen mucosa in the young calf. J Dairy Sci 1959;42:1600–5.
15. Harrison HN, Warner RG, Sander EG, et al. Changes in the tissue and volume of the stomachs of calves following the removal of dry feed or consumption of inert bulk. J Dairy Sci 1960;43:1301–12.
16. Warner, et al. The effect of various dietary factors on the development of the rumen. Proc Cornell Nutr Conf 1959;91–5.
17. Stobo IJF, Roy JHB, Gaston HJ. Rumen development in the calf. I. The effect of diets containing different proportions of concentrates to hay on rumen development. Br J Nutr 1966;20:171–92.
18. Warner RG. Nutritional factors affecting the development of a functional ruminant - a historical perspective. Proc Cornell Nutr Conf 1991;1–13.
19. Kertz A. F. 2021. Calf rumen development: Is roughage beneficial? Progressive Dairyman, January 13, 2021
20. National Research Council. Nutrient requirements of dairy cattle. 7th Revised Edition 2001.
21. Kramer M, Lund P, Weisbjerg MR. Rumen passage kinetics of forage- and concentrate-derived fiber in dairy cows. J Dairy Sci 2013;96:3163–76.
22. Counotte GH, van't Klooster AT, van der Kuilen J, et al. An analysis of the buffer system in the rumen of dairy cattle. J Anim Sci 1979;49:1536–44.

Moving?

Make sure your subscription moves with you!

To notify us of your new address, find your **Clinics Account Number** (located on your mailing label above your name), and contact customer service at:

Email: journalscustomerservice-usa@elsevier.com

800-654-2452 (subscribers in the U.S. & Canada)
314-447-8871 (subscribers outside of the U.S. & Canada)

Fax number: 314-447-8029

Elsevier Health Sciences Division
Subscription Customer Service
3251 Riverport Lane
Maryland Heights, MO 63043

*To ensure uninterrupted delivery of your subscription, please notify us at least 4 weeks in advance of move.

Printed and bound by CPI Group (UK) Ltd, Croydon, CR0 4YY

03/10/2024

01040482-0013